S-formula is t... ...

Health

Internal

body

cleaning

S-formula

India

Swamy sr

DEDICATED TO

EACH AND EVERY PERSON OF

WOLD.

My aim is to make the whole world

free from all diseases.

I want to see all the people of all

over the world happy and healthy

KEEP ALWAYS YOUR SEX

ORGANS STRONG

Internal body cleaning, written by S.R.Swamy

Published by NAVAYUGA PRAKASHANA,

Kathrekenahally, HIRIYUR Taluk,

KARNATAKA-INDIA – 577598

Swamysr90@gmail.com

Mobile: 9632559162

First Edition: 2017

Copies: 1000

Pages: 326

Price   : Rs. 500=00.

D.T.P: S.R.S, Kathrekenahalli, Hiriyur, Karnataka.

INTRODUCTION

Internal body cleaning - Internal body cleaning is done by Semen in our body. Semen is an organic fluid. Semen contains more than 200 chemicals. It will take all impurities which are not required for body to outside the body through urine, Latrine, Sweat, etc.

The semen is the energy to work all organs in our body. Semen is required for brain. Semen is required for reproduction. Semen is required for body cleaning. The use is your choice.

If you drink alcohol, chew tobacco, the semen stops all other works and start removing all impurities from tobacco or alcohol.

During this process lot of semen is wasted. All other development activities stops. Your body, brain destroyed.

So do not put any impurities in your body. If you put impurities semen will waste.

Use of semen is very big topic in our life. Lots of people do not know how to use semen of our body.

I done 33 years research on this matter and I am sharing my Knowledge. I am sure that this is real fact.

Semen is our body energy. Semen develops our body and mind throughout life.Semen is our body resistance. It will fight with harmful virus and Bacteria.

Semen keeps our body in good and healthy condition. Semen keeps our digestive system, Respiratory system, nerves system in good and perfect condition.

Semen produces sperm in male body and ovum in female body.Semen combine both sperm and ovum to form new baby. Semen takes all the energies from all the parts of male and female body.

Semen is an organic fluid. It contains more than 200 chemicals. It will make the baby to grow from day one to nine months in the mother stomach.

When the baby in stomach is able to produce semen by taking food , it will come out of mother stomach.

Semen develops nine months our body and mind in the stomach of mother. Semen develops our body from birth upto twenty five years in fully condition.

After the child birth upto twenty five years our body and mind is in growing stage, it is under process, during this time you should not waste semen. If you waste semen below twentyfive years, your development of body and mind stops.

Semen develops our body upto twenty five years and nourishes our body upto seventy five years.

After twenty five years , semen in our body develops new nerves, new layers in nerves, develops brain etc in our body.

You should not waste one drop of semen in your life. The man one who not waste semen throughout life is called Healthy man.

You use semen when you need baby.

Otherwise you should not waste single drop of semen. Loss of semen is injurious to health.

The speed of blood plays very important role in our body. The speed of blood is maintained by the semen in our body. As semen increases in our body , our blood speed increases. As the semen quantity decreases in our body, our speed of blood decreases.

There are lots of methods are there to waste semen is listed below. Due to continue waste of semen, the pressure inside our body is goes out with the semen. The pressure inside our body is lie force.

This force will be reduced by loss of semen. As this pressure decreases, the speed of blood goes down.

As the speed of blood goes down, your body will not work as per signals given by your brain.

Blood will not flow easily in your vans if the pressure reduces inside your body. Semen produces and maintains pressure inside our body.

Please donot waste semen and do not waste the pressure inside your body. Loss of semen is injurious to health. Due to loss of semen, loss of pressure, your brain, heart, vanes, respiratory system, digestive system, nervous system etc, all 79 organs will destroy slowly. And you will suffer lot of pain and diseases, finally you will die.

Please do not waste semen. save semen and enjoy the beautiful life.

All diseases are coming due to loss of semen only. Reason for loss of semen – how semen loss in our body.

The following are the reasons for the semen loss in

our body

If you think about sex matter, masturbation, cause more loss of semen.

If you drink alcohol , too much loss of semen occurs

If you use tobacco , it kills semen in your body, too much loss of semen

If you eat more salt in food, more spicy in food, it kills semen in your body.

Bad food kills semen in your body.

Semen is in the form of saliva juice in mouth, if you put saliva outside mouth, it is waste of semen

Semen is in the form of sweat, if you more sweat, it is the loss of semen.

Semen is in the form of tears, if you waste more tears, it is the symbol of loss of semen.

If you do more urine it is the loss of semen

If you do more latrine, it is the waste of semen

If you talk more, it is the loss of semen.

If you hear more noise it is loss of semen

If you talk more it is the loss of semen.

If you sleep more it is the loss of semen

If you eat more and more, it will cause loss of semen, and so on...

The s-formula says that, you please store more and more semen in your body.

Courage coming from our body semen, as the semen quantity increases in our body, our body become shining and charming. Loss of semen is loss of Courage. The secrete of Courage is semen. When semen quantity increases in your body , your Courage increases. When a semen quantity decreases in your body , your Courage decreases. So save semen in your body and increase your memory power.

Waste of one drop of semen is the waste of one drop of brain. Semen is food for Brain. If you lose semen you lose your brain. Brain is very important organ in our body. This book contains the importance of semen in every human life.

When the baby in the stomach of mother, it takes nine months to develop body in perfect condition. The baby less than nine months or eight months is not a perfect baby, there should be a lot of development of body is pending. So a perfect baby should be nine months or more.

In the same way, when the baby comes out of stomach of mother, it takes twenty five years to develop body in perfect condition. The man below twenty-five years is not a perfect man. So perfect man should be twenty five or more.

When a baby is in the stomach of its mother, the development of body and mind is done by semen.

When the baby come out of stomach of mother, the development of a body and mind up to twenty five years is done by semen.

If the baby in the stomach of mother, if the mother waste semen, the development of baby become very poor.

When the baby after coming out from the stomach of mother, if it waste semen within twenty five years, the development of body and mind become very poor.

If the mother wastes semen in her body, or if the baby waste semen within twenty five years, he is not a perfect man.

Perfect man means, a man one who not waste single drop of semen upto twenty five years he is called perfect man.

You read this book; it elaborates the importance of semen preservation in human body and negative effects of wasting semen. This book says in your life, you have checked with wasting semen, you have long life, please try just one year, with preserving semen, then you will know the meaning of life, you will know the difference. You will know the reason behind the successful personality. Actually life is experiment, if you do not succeed with one way; you should have to try with another way.

Vital energy is the essence of your body, preservation of it is the key to longevity of youthfulness. All worldly actions are performed through the body. If the body is weak and sickly, the mind becomes similarly afflicted. To attain success in any enterprise that both body and the mind are healthy and function in harmony and synchronicity.

Many young people, by wasting semen through uncontrolled sexual indulgence, they have lost mental, vital and physical energies with the result that their mind becomes sluggish, will power is lost and body becomes languid and sickly. Self realisation will remain a distant dream and they have somehow to drag along the remaining part of the life aimlessly.

Throughout history, great sages, saints and seers have stressed the paramount importance of S-formula for leading a noble and sublime life. Semen is thinned by its wastage, the more the wastage of semen, the more the body weakness.

The preservation of semen is the secrete of good health, longevity and of all success in the physical, mental, intellectual and spiritual planes. It is also true that one who preserves semen strictly is usually not afflicted by any disease.

By

S.R.Swamy jyothi, (S.R.S),Kathrekenahalli

S-FORMULA AUTHOR   -   S.R.S –

Education is the best friend. An educated person is respected everywhere. Education beats the beauty and the youth. Youth is not a time of life; it is a state of mind; it is not a matter of rosy cheeks, red lips and supple knees; it is a matter of the will, quality of the imagination, a vigour of the emotions; it is the freshness of the deep springs of life. There is a fountain of youth: it is your mind, your talents, the creativity you bring to your life and the lives of people you love. When you learn to tap this source, you will truly have defeated age.

Probably the happiest period in life most frequently is in middle age, when the eager passions of youth are cooled, and the infirmities of age not yet begun;

as we see that the shadows, which are at morning and evening so large, almost entirely disappear at midday. What sadden me is the corruption of youth and beauty, and the loss of soul, which is only replaced by money. Education is not a tool for development - individual, community and the nation. It is the foundation for our future. It is empowerment to make choices and emboldens the youth to chase their dreams. Good habits formed at youth make all the difference. Keep true to the dreams of your youth. In youth we learn; in age we understand. Youth is the spirit of adventure and awakening. It is a time of physical emerging when the body attains the vigour and good health that may ignore the caution of temperance. Youth is a period of timelessness when the horizons of age seem too distant to be noticed. The youth is the hope of our future. Forty is the old age of youth; fifty the youth of old age.

The greatest wealth and strength of any nation is its youth. The future of a nation lies in the hands of its posterity. The quality of its youth determines the kind of future, the nation will have. Therefore, if we want to ensure a bright future for our country, we first need to strengthen and empower our youth. The youth of any nation and society are its potential energy. They are the powerhouse and storehouse of infinite energy. They are the ones who are the pride of the nation. It is the youth which brings laurels to their country. The best and the first and foremost way to strengthen our youth are to provide them education. Not just any kind of education, but the right kind of education which makes them scientific, logical, open-minded, self respecting, responsible, honest and patriotic. Without these virtues being developed, our youth cannot walk in the desired way and they will remain in a deep slumber of complacency.

Our youths are spoiling like anything, nobody is teaching our youths properly,

Our government, our scientists, our doctors, our swamijis, our so many brilliant officers, are not telling the youths, to save semen, Teenagers are spoiling like anything, I will give you some evidences about s-formula, Genius people talking about courage, but, they are not telling the secrete how to get courage, where is that courage, Genius peoples talking about health, but, they are not telling how to get health, In the same way lot of good characters, good things they are telling, but, they fail to tell the secrete how to get all these, S-formula is the only one thing everything it gives to us, Do not sit quite, please help rural peoples, innocents, uneducated persons this secrete, Please help our people, help our youths, help our country, Let us do all s-formula, and become more powerful.

Many teens suffer from mental health issues in response to the pressures of society and social problems they encounter. Some of the key mental health issues seen in teens are: depression, eating disorders, and drug abuse. S-formula is the one and only way to prevent these health issues from occurring such as communicating well with a teen suffering from mental health issues. Mental health can be treated and be attentive to teens' behaviour,

-S.R.S –

ABOUT S-FORMULA

To bring peace in the world, s-formula is made. S-formula means save semen. Semen - the foundation of a male & female body.

Semen is like electrical current in our body. Semen keeps our body, hot in cold region, cold in hot region.

The conservation of semen is very essential to strength of body and mind.

Semen is an organic fluid, seminal fluid.

Look younger, think cleverer, live longer, if you save semen.

20

Veerya, dhatu, shukra or semen is life.

Virginity is a physical, moral, and intelluctual safe guard to young man.

Semen is the most powerful energy in the world.

One who has master of this art is the master of all.

Semen is truely a precious jewel.

A greek philosopher told that only once in his life time.

Conservation of seminal energy is s-formula.

As you think, so you become.

Semen is marrow to your bones, food to your brain, oil to your joints, and sweetness to your breath.

Chastity no more injures the body and the soul. Self discipline is better than any other line of conduct.

A healthy mind lives in a healthy body.

If children are ruined, the nation is ruined.

S-formula is the art of living, it is the art of life, and it is the way of life.

The person one who knows s-formula; he is the master of all arts.

Whatever the problems, diseases comming from loss of semen, can be rectified by only by saving semen.

Semen produces semen & semen kills semen.

Always save semen, store semen; protect semen from birth to death.

Semen once you lost that will not come back – lost is lost.

Loss of semen causes your life waste.

Quality of your life says the quality of your semen.

Use semen only when you need baby.

Waste of one drop of semen is the waste of one drop of brain.

Keep always the level of semen more than that normal level in your body.

All diseases will attack due to loss of semen only.

You do any physical exercise only if you are healthy.

. Prevention is better than cure.

Semen is a pure blood and food for all cells of your body.

Semen once you wasted can not be regained. Lost is lost.

Waste persons are wasting lot of semen.

You reject marriages, if you waste semen.

Considering all the youths, the entire nations, the entire world, i did research.

My name is S.R.Swamy, a civil engineering graduate, born in 1968 AD, hiriyur talluk, Karnataka state. I am a karate master, yoga master, sanjeevini vidye panditha. I done 35 years research on god and found the secrete of god. I done 35 years research on health and found the secrete of health. I invented S-formula.

Today January 2017 AD, we are presenting S-formula to the world. S-formula is not a medicine but it is a type of meditation. It is knowledge based training. S-formula solves all your problems, diseases etc.

The growth and development of human body is slowly reducing day by day. We must stop this. If all are following s-formula from today, they will grow fast and they will lift mountain, otherwise if they are not following from today, they will walk on water in future days.

S-formula is yoga. It is the real youth power. It is a code word.

By

S.R.Swamy jyothi (S.R.S), Kathrekenahalli

Value of semen

The human seed, of course, contain all essential elements necessary to create another human being when it is united with ovum. In a pure and orderly life this matter (semen) is reabsorbed, it goes back into circulation ready to form the finest brain, nerve and muscular tissues. Whenever the seminal secretions are conserved and thereby reabsorbed into the system, it goes towards enriching the blood and strengthening the brain.

An analysis of both brain cells and semen shows great similarities; both are very high in phosphorus, sodium, magnesium and chlorine. The sex glands and the brain cells are intimately connected physiologically but are adversaries in the sense that they are both competing for the same nutritional elements from the identical blood stream. In this sense the brain and the sexual organs are also competitors in using bodily energy and nutrition's.

25

There are only so many nutrients in our blood stream. Our body can only assimilate limited quantities of nutrients in a given period of time. Phosphorus for example is required in both the thinking and reproductive process, still your body can only assimilates finite or limited quantities of phosphorus from the diet to meet these demands in a twenty-four hours period. If most nutrition's in your blood are going into meeting demands of your gonads and being ejaculated, there will be a little left over to meet nutritional demands of the rest of your body and brain. The energy of our body is most potent when used in one direction.

The loss of energy due to excessive ejaculation is a slow and subtle process that most men do not usually notice until it is too late. After countless episodes, a deterioration of your body sets in. As a man gets older, he may rationalise this lack of energy and loss of sexual vigour on his age. He is only too happy to continue pumping out his semen, sometimes even paying for the privilege and accelerating his deterioration.

The precise word for it should be going, because everything, the erecting, vital energy, millions of live sperms/ovum, hormones, nutrients, even a little of the man's personality goes away. It is a great scarifies for the man, spiritually, mentally and physically.

Semen nourishes the physical body, the heart and the intellect. Nature puts the most valuable ingredients in the seed in all forms of life, in order to provide for continuation of the species, and the fluid semen, a man discharges during sexual relations containing the human seed. The human seed, of course, contains all essential elements necessary to create another human being, when it is united with ovum. It contains forces capable of creating life. Wasting of semen is very bad for health; it makes you dry, loose, skinny, weak and impotent day by day.

The strength of the body, the light of the eyes and the entire life of the man is slowly being lost by too much loss of semen. We to conserve seminal fluid for nourishing, improving and perfecting our body and brain, when reproduction is not mutually desired.

All the waste of spermatic secretions, whether voluntary or involuntary, is a direct waste of the life force. The conservation of semen is essential to strength of body, vigour of mind and keenness of intellect.

Falling of semen brings death, preservation of semen gives life. If the semen is lost, the man become nervous, then the mind also cannot work properly, the man become fickle minded, there is a mental weakness.

One ejaculation of semen will lead to wastage of wealth of energy. However much semen are able to retain, you will receive in that proportion grater wisdom, improves action, higher spirituality and increased knowledge.

Semen is a beautiful, sparking word, when reflecting on it one's mind is filled with grand, great, majestic, beautiful and powerful emotions. It is the secrete of magnetic personality.

If you store and protect semen in your body, you will acquire the power to get whatever you want. If semen remains in the body, it is the essence of vitality, their descriptions of the body glowing with energy of semen. Grasp fully the importance and value of semen, vital essence of life.

Semen is all power, all money, God in motion; it is god, Dynamic will, Atmabal, Thought, Intelligence and Consciousness. Therefore preserve this vital fluid very very carefully. Semen is our body power, Life force, Stamina, it is our energy, and it is our memory power, our courage, mental power.

The best blood in the body goes to form semen. It is essential to strength of body, vigour of mind and keenness of intellect.

Semen loss is harmful. Seminal fluid is considered as an elixir of life in the physical and mystical sense. Its preservation guarantees health, longevity and super natural powers. Conservation of semen results in the emergence of a charismatic power in the body. The science of seminal conservation allows you to conserve seminal fluid for nourishing, improving and perfecting our body and brain when reproduction is not mutually desired.

The seminal fluid is a viscid, proteinnaceous fluid; it is rich in potassium, iron, lecithin, vitamin E, protease, spermine, albumen, phosphorous, calcium and other organic minerals and vitamins.

Mahatma Gandhi in 1959 told that the strength of the body, the light of the eyes and the entire life of a man is slowly being lost by too much loss of semen, the vital fluid.

How Semen Formed

Semen is formed out of food. The formation of semen form is very lengthy process. Food is filtered seven times, so called s-formula. Food will be converted into semen in seven stages. Semen is required to convert food into semen. Semen produces semen. Semen is produced by semen. Blood filtered seven times so that semen is a pure blood.

Out of Food formed Chyle (Rasa)

Out of Chyle comes Blood

Out of Blood comes Flesh

Out of Flesh comes Fat

Out of Fat comes Bone

Out of Bone comes Bone marrow

Out of Bone marrow comes Semen.

Statement as how semen is formed through seven stages proves. Only 20 grams semen is produced from that a man consumes in nearly 35 days.

From 32000 grams food approximately 11153 grams Chyle is formed.

From 11153 grams of Chyle approximately 3887 grams of Blood is formed.

From 3887 grams of Blood approximately 1355 grams of Flesh is formed.

From 1355 grams of Flesh approximately 472grams of Fat is formed.

From 472 grams of Fat approximately 164 grams of Bone is formed.

From 164 grams of Bone approximately 57 grams of Bone marrow is formed.

From 57 grams of Bone marrow approximately 20 grams of Semen is formed.

The semen is true of your body. A man cannot think or perform his best when much of this energy and bloods nutrients are expended in the discharge of semen. Not only a proper diet necessary to keep arteries clean, so blood can flow freely to all vital organs as well as your corpora cavernous penis, but also to replenish body chemistry.

Just as a bees collect honey in the honeycomb drop by drop, so also, the cells collect semen drop by drop from the blood.

Semen contains ingredients like Fructose, sugar, water, ascorbic acid, citric acid, enzymes, proteins, phosphate and bicarbonate buffers zinc. Seminal fluid contains fatty acids, fructose and proteins to nourish the sperm and ovum.

If semen wasted, it leaves him effeminate, weak and physically debilitated and prone to sexual irritation and disordered function, a wretched nervous system, epilepsy and various other diseases and death.

A typical ejaculation fills up about one teaspoon. Since sperm makeup only one percent of semen, the rest of ninety-nine percent is composed of over two hundred separate proteins, vitamins, minerals, etc.It takes seventy four days for sperm to be produced and fully matured to be ready for ejaculation. So any sperm that you ejaculate today is at least seventy four days old.

The semen can be extracted by the testicles and reabsorbed to strengthen the body and brain. Semen is a mysterious secretion that is able to create a living body. Semen itself is a living substance, it is life itself. Therefore when it leaves man it takes a portion of his own life.

Chemical Composition of semen.

Semen is composed of over two hundred separate proteins, as well as vitamins and minerals including vitaminC. Calcium, chlorine, citric acid, fructose, lactic acid, magnesium, nitrogen, phosphorous, potassium, sodium, vitamin B12 and Zinc. Levels of these compounds vary depending on age, weight and lifestyle habits like diet and exercise.

The chemical composition of semen is as follows.

Chemical name – mg per 100ml

Ammonia – 2mg per 100ml

Ascorbic acid – 12.80

Ash – 9.90

Calcium – 25

Carbon di oxide – 54 ml

Chloride – 155

Cholesterol - 80

Citric acid – 376

Creatine – 20

Ergothioneine – trace

Fructose – 224

Glutathione – 30

Glyceryl phoryl choline – 54-90

Inositol – 50.57

Lactic acid – 35

Magnesium – 14

Nitrogen no protein (total) – 913

Phosphorus, acid soluble – 57

Inorganic – 11

Lipids – 6

Total lipids – 112

Phosphoryl choline – 250-380

Potassium – 89

Pyruvic acid – 29

Sodium – 281

Sorbitol – 10

Vitamin B12 – 300-600 ppg

Sulphur – 3% (of ash)

Urea – 72

Uric acid – 6

Zinc – 14

Copper – 006-024

The chemical compositions of sperm that benefit the body are as follows.

Calcium – This composition is very useful for bones and teeth and even to maintain muscle and nerve function.

Citric acid – Useful to prevent blood clotting in the body.

Creatine – useful to increase energy and formation of muscle and also acts as a fat burner.

Ergothionine – Functions as protection of skin from DNA damage.

Glutathione – This is very useful as cancer prevention drugs. Prevent blood clotting during surgery and increase the efficiency chemotherapy drugs.

Inositol – Functions to prevent hair loss.

Lactic acid – Serve as a material for burns and surgical wounds.

Lipid – Functions as a fat burner.

Pyruvic acid – Functioning as fertilising.

Sorbitol – Used by pharmacists as a material to overcome constipation.

Urea – Serves to remove excess nitrogen in the body.

Uric acid – Useful for the prevention of diabetes but most uric acid would be caused disease gout etc.

Sulphur – Useful for smoothing the skin.

Vitamin B12 – as an addition to stamina.

Fructose – Can serve as a digestive sugar in the body, which is very useful for the prevention of diabetes. Most fructose is also dangerous because it can cause gout.

Zinc – Useful as an acne drug.

All of the above substances are very important substances, which are very beneficial for the body and are used for a variety of healing medicines.

Study of semen

Several studies reveal that semen responds and is impacted by what they eats. What they eat daily plays very important role in the health of their semen.

During the process of ejaculation sperm passes through the ejaculatory ducts and mixes with fluids from the seminal vesicles, the prostate and the bulbourethral glands to form the semen. Seminal plasma of human contains a complex range of organic and inorganic constituents.

1992 world health organisation report described normal human semen is having a volume of 2 ml or grater. PH of 7.2 – 8.0, sperm concentration of 20x (10)6spermatazoa / ml or more, sperm count of 40x (10)6 spermatozoa per ejaculate or more.

The average reported physical and chemical properties of human semen were as follows

Property - per 100 ml – in average volume (3.40 ml)

Calcium (mg) – 27.60 – 0.938

Chloride (mg) – 142 – 4.83

Citrate (mg) – 528 – 18.00

Fructose (mg) – 272 – 9.2

Glucose (mg) – 102 – 3.47

Lactic acid (mg) – 62 – 2.11

Magnesium (mg) – 11 – 0.374

Potassium (mg) – 109 – 3.71

Protein (g) – 5.04 – 0.171

Sodium (mg) – 300 – 10.20

Urea (mg) – 45 – 1.53

Zinc (mg) – 16.50 – 0.561

Semen quality is a measure of the ability of semen to accomplish fertilization. The volume of semen ejaculate varies but is generally one teaspoon full or less.

In ancient Greece, Greek philosophy Aristotle remarked on the importance of semen. There is a direct connection between food and semen, food and physical growth. He warns against engaging in sexual activities at too early an age, this will affect the growth of their bodies. The transformation of nourishment into semen does not drain the body of needed material. The region around the eyes was the region of the head. SEMEN IS A DROP OF BRAIN.

Women were believed to have their own version, which was stored in the womb, and released during climax.

Semen is considered a form of miasma and ritual purification was to be practised after its discharge. One drop of semen is manufactured out of forty drops of blood according to the medical science. According to Ayurveda it is elaborated out of eighty drops of blood.

Semen is a natural anti-depressant. Semen elevates your mood and even reduces suicidal thoughts.

Semen reduces anxiety, it boasts anti anxiety hormones like oxytocin, serotonin and progesterone.

Semen improves the quality of your sleep; it contains melatonin, a sleep inducing agent.

Semen increases the energy, it improves mental alertness. It even improves memory. It reduces pain.

Semen improves cardio health and prevents preeclampsia, which causes dangerously high blood pressure during pregnancy.

Semen prevents morning sickness, but only if it is the same semen that caused your pregnancy.

Semen slows down the aging process of your skin and muscle. It contains a healthy portion of zinc, which is an anti oxidant.

Semen improves mental alertness.

I done 35 years research, study and analysis on god and found the secrete of god .i done 35 years research and analysis about health and invented the secrete of health. I invented s-formula.

S-formula means save semen, store semen, protect semen in your body. Do not waste the semen from your body. Do not make any activities which cause loss of semen in your body. Always involve in the activities which supports to save semen in your body. Save semen always throughout your life.

s-formula is a code word - for common people to talk in public. (semen means male semen and female semen in all humans). S-formula is also called as celibacy, brahmachrya, chastity. Semen is also called as veerya, dhathu, shukra, etc in many languages.

S-formula is the vital energy that supports your life. It gives strength, power, energy, courage to your life. It shines your sparking eyes. It beems in your shining cheeks. It is a great treasure for you. It gives colour and vitality to the human body and its different organs. It develops strong mind and strong body. It is the real vitality in man. It gives you more strength and good health.

The basic secrete of human power is s-formula. If you follow s-formula you will become more powerful and rich. It is the real power of a man.

S-formula is not a medicine but it is a type of meditation. It is knowledge based training. It is a foundation for all life. It is a world dharma, it is like a god, it is the foundation for all dharma's, all religions, all shasta's, all sampradayas. It is the super natural power that surviving the whole world.

S-formula is the secrete of health, it is the real spiritual power, real body power, it is our internal body power, it is our internal body resistance, it is the secrete of beauty.

S-formula controls angry and gives peace of mind, it also controls the people becoming mad, it controls corruption activities, poor will become rich, good citizens are born from s-formula.

S-formula is the power of any nation, it is the anti corruption weapon, it will cure all diseases, it makes your bones strong and hard, it will increases power of your sex organs; it will increases your health and wealth. Good characters are born by s-formula.

A man will lift the mountain if he follows s-formula. A man will walk on water if he not follows s-formula, in future 5000 years onwards.

S-formula is the art of living, it is the way of life, it is the secrete of life. One who has master of this art is the master of all. Semen is very precious content of the body; it comes out from bone marrow that lies concealed inside the bones. Semen is formed in a subtle state in all the cells of the body. This vital fluid of a man carried back and diffused through his system make him manly strong, brave, and heroic. Semen is considered a precious material formed by the distillation of blood. Semen is the quintessence of blood, it is an organic fluid, it is a hidden treasure in man, it is also known as seminal fluid. Semen contains forces capable of creating life; it is the vital energy that supports your life.

Herbal medical science, founder of ayurveda, dhanvantari thought that semen is truely a precious jewel. It is the most effective medicine which destroys diseases, decay and death.

For attaining peace, brightness, memory, knowledge, health and self realisation. One should observe the way of semen preservation, the highest knowledge, greatest strength, highest dharma. You can see how precious the semen is.

The spermatic secretion in man is continuous, it must either be expelled or be reabsorbed into the system, it goes towards enriching the blood and strengthening the brain.

According to dhanvantari, the sexual energy is transmitted into spiritual energy by pure thoughts. It is the process of controlling of sex energy, conserving it, then diverting it into higher channel and finally converting it into spiritual energy or shakti.

Shakti cause attractive personality, the person is outstanding in his works; his speech is impressive and thrilling. This stored up energy can be utilised for divine contemplation and spiritual pursuits, self realisation.

Assuming that an ordinary man consumes thirty two kilograms of food in forty days, yielding eight hundred grams of blood, which intern will yield only twenty grams of semen over a period of one month. One month accumulation of semen is discharged in one sexual intercourse.

Sex is not an entertainment. If a man leads a life of s-formula, even in householder life and has copulation for the sake of pregnancy only, he can bring healthy, intelligent, strong, beautiful and self sacrificing children.

There is a great injustice being done to the youth at present time. They face attack from all sides, which is sex stimulating. On the basis of the science of corruption founded by misleading psycho analyst, then god alone can save the celibacy of the youth and chastity of the married couples. Lack of self control give rise to diseases, mental illness.

semen gives solution to the problem of suppressing desires. Sex undoubtedly leads to spiritual downfall. Self control is the essential to attain super conscious. This is indian philosophy.

Many ordinary people become yogis by following the principles of indian psychology founded by sage pathanjali. Many are trading this path and many will follow it.

Pre marital sex and masturbation, unethical and unnatural sex causes psychiatry, neuroses. They are unconscious enmity against parents, bisexuality, incest drives, latent home security, inverted love, hate relationships, murderous death wishes, calamitous sibling rivalries, unseen hatred of every description, spastic colon, near continuous depressive moods, neurasthenia, and homo sexual tendencies, bad temper, migraines, constipation, travel phobias, infected sinuses, fainting sleeps and hostile drives of hate and murder, victims of superstitions, magical numbers and childish gullibility.

If sexual urge is not controlled, excessive sexual intercourse drains the energy enormously, persons are physically, mentally and morally debilitated by wasting the seminal power. You experience much exhaustion and weakness.

Prevention of seminal energy is the vital subject for those who want success in marital or spiritual life. It is essential for strong body and sharp brain.

Maharishi pathanjali has stated in his yoga, one who has accomplished perpetual sublimation of semen through yoga, he become all powerful. Through celibacy the impossible become possible. The gain of fame, wealth and other material things is assured to the s-formula.

A greek philosopher told that only once in his life time.

A house holder can have copulation with his legal wife. Priceless human life is wasted in sexual indulgence but sexual desires are never satiated. One, who wastes his semen for sexual pleasure, finally attains despaired, weakness and death.

In the present day world (2017 ad), unfortunately people read pornographic literature, view sex films on television and in theatres, view blue films in privacy, as a result we see all around us. The number of physical, mental and moral wrecks increasing every day. Many times such people indulge in unnatural sex.masturbation or homosexual tendency lead them to wastage of seminal energy many times a week. They may discharge seminal energy in bad dreams.

Due to excessive loss of semen, persons are physically, mentally and morally debilitated. The evil after effects that follow the loss of seminal energy are dangerous. The body and mind refuse to work energetically. Due to excessive loss of semen pain in the testes, enlargement of testes develops; impotency comes for test ices cannot produce semen with normal sperm count. Therefore practice of s-formula is always commendable.

By the practice of s-formula, longevity, glory, strength, vigour, knowledge, wealth, undying fame, virtues and devotion to truth increases.

But if you not practice s-formula, you will suffer from lack of thinking power, restless of mind, nervous breakdown, debility, pain in testes, fickle mindedness, and weak kidneys. Pain in head and joints, pain in back, palpitation of heart, gloominess, loss of memory, number of diseases like anaemia.

Through away sexual desires which destroy your strength, intelligence and health. Do not involve in any activities that wastes your seminal energy.

Atharva veda says that one who not led a life of celibacy, the lust is the cause of diseases; it is the cause of death. It makes one walk with tottering steps. It causes mental debility and retardation. It destroys health, vitality and physical well being. It burns or dhatus namely chyle, blood, flesh, fat, bone, bone marrow, semen. It pollutes the purity of mind.

S-formula is an inspiring uplifting word. S-formula practice is one who is married or unmarried, who does not indulge in sex, who shuns the company of women and men sex.

The preservation of seminal energy for both the sex is considered to be s-formula. Preservation of semen is only the final goal. The ultimate goal of human life is to attain self knowledge. They expect nothing from the world. Conservation of seminal energy is s-formula. The realisation of one's owns self. S-formula is absolute freedom from sexual desires and thoughts.

The more luxurious of life one leads, the more difficult it becomes for them to preserve their seminal energy. Simple living is a sign of greatness.

Learn to follow the lives of great saintly souls. Do not be impressed by the life style of egoistic people.

Physician says that eat five hundred grams of food in a day. This much is enough for nutrition of the body. If any take more, it is a burden on digestive system. It reduces the longevity of life. Generally people stuff the stomach with delicacies to enjoy the taste. Stuffing the stomach is highly deleterious, but they die early. Such indulgence of the sense of the taste will also lead to frequent discharge of semen in dreams. Thus one will gradually become a victim of diseases and ruin.

Solid food is easily digested if it takes when the breathing mainly takes place through right nostril. Whenever you take any liquid food, make sure that left nostril is open. Beware do not take any liquid when the right nostril is open.

Do not overload the stomach at night. Overloading is the direct cause of nocturnal emission. Take easily digestible light food at night.

Do not take very hot food or heavy food as they cause diseases. Hot food and hot tea weaken the teeth and gums. They make the semen watery.

Cooked, canned, fried, processed, irradiated, barbecued, micro waved, de germinated, preserved, chemical zed, homogenized, pasteurized and otherwise devitalized foods are not the best materials to be converted into healthy tissues, blood and vital organs needed for vigorous health – and certainly not to meet the demands of an active sexual life.

Things fried in oil or ghee, over cooked foods, spicy foods, chutneys, chillies, meat, fish, egg, garlic, onion, liquor, sour articles and stale food preparations should be avoided for they stimulate the sexual organs.

Thoroughly chew the food. No strenuous work should be done immediately after meals. Take water in the middle or 30 to 60 minutes after the meal. Eating after midnight is not good. One should never take warm milk at night before going to bed. It usually causes wet dreams.

Use spinach, green leafy vegetables, milk, butter, ghee, buttermilk, fresh fruits for preserving seminal energy.

Never stops the urge to answer the calls of nature. A loaded bladder is the cause of wet dreams.

You should take recourse to occasional fasting. One should fast in accordance to his capacity. Overeating and excessive fasting both are danger to health. Fasting controls passion and destroys sexual excitement.

A healthy mind lives in a healthy body. One should regularly practice physical exercises early in the morning. The purpose of exercise is to keep it free from diseases, body and mind should be healthy.

By doing any type of physical exercises, production of semen in your body increases, as semen increases, your sex organs become strong. Always keep your sex organs strong, this is the secrete of health. Do not waste semen at this stage.

Strong will helps in preservation of seminal energy. Will is the powerful enemy of passion. Develop dynamic will power, as you think, so you become.

Some memorable statements

Semen is marrow to your bones, food to your brain, oil to your joints, and sweetness to your breath.

Chastity no more injures the body and the soul. Self discipline is better than any other line of conduct.

Virginity is a physical, moral and intellectual safeguard to young man.

The energy that is wasted during one sexual intercourse is the energy that is utilized in the mental work for three days. Semen is very precious vital fluid. Do not waste this energy. Preserve it with great care, you will have wonderful vitality. Semen transmuted into spiritual energy or shakti.

Most of your ailments are due to excessive seminal wastage. Semen is the most powerful energy in the world. Self realisation is the goal.

When this energy semen is once wasted, it can never be recouped by any other means. You must try your level best to preserve every drop although you are a married man.

Excessive sexual intercourse drains the energy enormously. Young man do not realise the value of the vital fluid. They waste this dynamic energy.

He who wasted the semen becomes easily irritable, losses his balance of mind, become furious. He behaves improperly. He does not know what he is exactly doing; he will do anything he likes. He will insult his parents, guru and respectable persons.

Preservation of semen, divine power, leads to the attainment of strong will power, good behaviour and spiritual exaltation.

Those who have lost much of their semen become very cruel, criminal, little thing upset their minds. They become the slaves of anger, jealousy, laziness and fear, their sense is not in under control, they do foolish acts. Bodily and mental strength gets diminished day by day.

Semen once lost is lost forever, never repair the loss completely.

Children's are the invaluable assets to the nation. If children are ruined, the nation is ruined. In order to save the nation, children should be saved from sex abuse. In order to build the character of school-going children and college students, they should be provided and encouraged to read the book of s-formula or like this book. So that they can know the glory of value of semen. By practicing s-formula, become brilliant and promising students. This is our moral duty. It is the moral duty of our government. Children's should be protected from drug addiction, exiting films and blue films.

Forty meals give rise to one drop of blood. Forty drop of blood gives rise to one drop of bone marrow. Forty drops of bone marrow give rise to one drop of semen. So semen is considered a precious material.

S-formula improves the condition of your semen. The semen nourishes the brain. Semen retained in the body goes upwards to nourish the brain. Semen retention is very valuable for both spiritual and mental health. If semen is drying up makes one old. Semen is the real elixir of youth.

Sperm or ovum is the end product of all digestions and essential ointment. Semen loss occurs through masturbation, results in mental illness. Semen is derived from the whole body, both parents created semen. Both the parents produce semen and contribute to their children.

S-formula is the art of living, it is the art of life, and it is the way of life. One who has mastered this art is the master of all. S-formula is the secrete of life.

All the common people of all over world must follow s-formula and must know the value of s-formula.

S-formula is a code word. Each and every citizen of country must communicate, talk, and discuss one by one to save semen.

S-formula means save semen

S, means semen

S, means seven dhathus

S, means seven stages of semen formation

S, is very popular word, that each and every citizen of world knows

S-formula is considered as the consolidated meaning of this whole book. In each and every house all the members should talk about the value of semen using this code word. If anybody express s-formula from his mouth, it is understood that he knows the value of semen. Do all the daily activities in your life by using s-formula, your life become beautiful.

The person one who knows s-formula; he is the master of all arts.

Some theory says that

Theory-1 -production of seminal fluids among these 3 glands is thought to be regulated based on need; however there does appear to be a constant, nominal production of fluid in these glands as well. In other words, the more often ejaculation occurs, the more fluid these glands will produce to attempt to keep the average volume of semen ejaculated at about 2.5ml - 5.0ml, or about 1-2 teaspoons. All three glands are thought to be able to reabsorb any excess fluid produced but not ejaculated, however this is only theory.

Theory-2-another theory is that the glands only produce what is needed to fill their storage capacities, and then stop producing until needed again after an ejaculation.

Theory-3-a third theory kind of combines these first two, with the thought that these glands reabsorb excess fluid to some extent, but production of new fluid is constant at some nominal level, with the ability to increase production based on need.

But the constant nominal production may exceed the reabsorption capacity of the glands, leading to a gradual build-up of seminal fluid, and eventual ejaculation through a nocturnal emission (wet dream) or a spontaneous ejaculation.

This theory that semen comes from the body is an ayurveda understanding wherein different materials of the body "distil" to form purer substances which are then extracted by the testicles as semen. The fact that semen comes from the testicles is no big discovery. The value of semen was stressed by ancient philosophers & doctors.

The basic principles of ayurveda involve a metaphysical understanding of the elements. The bodies tissues are divided into seven: rasa (plasma), rakta   (blood), mamsa   (muscle), meda   (fat tissues), asthi   (bone), majja (marrow), shukra   (semen).

The semen can be extracted by the testicles and reabsorbed to strengthen the body and brain. Semen is a mysterious secretion that is able to create a living body. Semen itself is living substance.

It is life itself. Therefore, when it leaves man, it takes a portion of his own life.a living thing cannot be put to laboratory tests, without first killing it. The scientist has no apparatus to test it.

God has provided the only test to prove its precious nature, viz., the womb. The very fact that semen is able to create life is proof enough that it is life itself.

What important people says

Dr. Nicole says: "it is a medical and physiological fact that the best blood in the body goes to form the elements of reproduction in both the sexes.

Dr. Dio louis thinks that the conservation of this element is essential to strength of body, vigour of mind and keenness of intellect.

Another writer, dr. E.p. Miller, says: all waste of spermatic secretions, whether voluntary or involuntary, is a direct waste of the life force. It is almost universally conceded that the choicest element of the blood enters into the composition of the spermatic secretion.

One ejaculation of semen will lead to wastage of a wealth of energy. This belief can be traced back to the holy scriptures (sushruta samhita, 1938; charak samhita, 1949; gandhi, 1957; kuma sutra, 1967).

One ejaculation of semen will lead to wastage of a wealth of energy. It is being propagated by the lay and pseudoscientific literature (mishra, 1962;

chand, 1968) and has fascinated many scientific investigators..." (malhotra and wig, 1975: 526) "(bottero, 1991: 306).

However much semen you are able to retain, you will receive in that proportion greater wisdom, improves action, higher spirituality and increased knowledge. Moreover, you will acquire the power to get whatever you want. (yogacharya bhagwandev 1992: 15) "[alter, 1997: 280].

Semen! What a beautiful, sparkling word! When reflecting on it one's mind is filled with grand, great, majestic, beautiful, and powerful emotions. [shastri n.d.[a]:10]"[alter, 1997: 284].

A large segment of the general public from all socioeconomic classes believes that semen loss is harmful. Seminal fluid is considered an elixir of life in the physical and mystical sense. Its preservation guarantees health, longevity, and supernatural powers" (malhotra and wig, 1975: 519).

Natural emission, or svapna dosh (dream error), is given special consideration by all authors. Kariraj jagannath shastri devotes his whole book to the subject, and because of its 'involuntary' nature, calls svapna dosh the worst of all 'personal diseases'" (alter, 1997: 287).

The master of taoist philosophy, dr. Stephen chang wrote: "when the average male ejaculates, he loses about one tablespoon of semen.according to scientific research, the nutritional value of this amount of semen is equal to that of two pieces of new york steak, ten eggs, six oranges, and two lemons combined.that includes proteins, vitamins, minerals, amino acids, everything… ejaculation is often called 'coming'.

Edwin flatto is a retired doctor living in florida and has been an nhf member since the 1950s. He is a graduate of the university of miami and the escuela homeopathic de allos estudios de guadalajara (medico homeopatico). Over the years ed has written 16 books on health, including, "super potency at any age", "miracle exercise that can save your life", and "home birth- step by step instructions". He is currently gold's gym instructor, has a son age 7, and has won four gold medals in the senior olympics. Order his book called "super potency at any age".

In nietzsche's notes (1880-1881) he writes: "the reabsorption of semen by the blood is the strongest nourishment and, perhaps more than any other factor, it prompts the stimulus of power, the unrest of all forces toward the overcoming of resistances, the thirst for contradiction and resistance. Nietzsche's did not mean reabsorption of semen by the blood thro digestion (oral sex). There is a hermit belief that by practising certain spiritual exercises one can redirect the sexual power into spiritual/intellectual/physical energy.the feeling of power has so far mounted highest in abstinent priests and hermits.

As for this theory on reabsorption of sperm, "sperm is full of protein". Also would have thought that some mysterious component of sperm capable of enhancing the mind in any way, somebody amongst the hordes of scientists performing research in the world today would have discovered it.

The effect may result in either very high intellectual/physical power or outright lunacy if gone wrong.! Modern science may interpret this as controlling associated hormones for good/bad. The scientists of old have put great value upon the vial fluid and they have insisted upon its strong transmutation into the highest form of energy for the befit of society."

Mahatma ghandi, 1959"the strength of the body, the light of the eyes, and the entire life of the man is slowly being lost by too much loss of the vital fluid."

Jewish code of lawssec. Orach chaim.ch. 240; parag. 14"the stuff of the sexual life is the stuff of art; if it is expended in one channel it is lost for the other.

Havelock ellis"i am quite willing to believe in the correctness of the regimens you recommend...and i do not doubt all of us would do better if we followed your maxims."

Eminent european medical men also support the statement of the yogins of india.

What happiness you get, by doing loss of semen, 100 times more than that happiness you will get in storing semen. When you store the semen, you feel lot of pressure on your sex organ, 24 hours, 365 days you feel happy. Save semen, and enjoy more happiness in your life.

Lot of people making money by selling products which cause loss of semen, do not spoil your life and do not make them rich by sacrificing your life.

You start storing semen, lot of marriage proposals you will get. By storing semen in your body, you are looking very attractive, charming, marrying people likes only attractive and charming. Save semen and enjoy marriage.

All civilized persons developing their life by implementing s-formula, without knowing that, this is s-formula. But lot of uncivilized citizens, suffering problems in their life, without following s-formula, but they do not know what s-formula is. Please everyone try to know the value of s-formula.s-formula is equal to god.

Benefits of s-formula

Benifits of s-formula is as follows – if you adopt and implement s-formula in your life, your whole body is glowing, free from all diseases and weakness in the body. Rose colour to the skin. Kills and reduces angry and increases peace of mind. It controls the growth and development of the body. Hairs remain black and no hair fall occurs. Free from eye sight problems. All joints and nerves become strong. The back bone will become very strong. You will get good health. Your face, eyes and chins will become shining and looks very attractive. Increasing of physical power and mental power. You will become highly courage; brave, highly intelligent and highly brilliant. You will get whatever you want. It increases yourself confidence, power and energy for perfecting your body and mind. You will be free from corruption mind, criminal mind. Poor will become rich; you will be free from poverty.

Whatever the problems, diseases comming from loss of semen, can be rectified by only by saving semen. There is no any medicine for this.

Semen produces semen & semen kills semen.

Always save semen, store semen; protect semen from birth to death.

Banana plant takes one year to make banana, it it impossible to create a banana manually in the laboratory. In the same way, our body will take thirty five days to make semen from food. It is impossible to make semen in the laboratory. It is produced and manufactured inside our body only. It is not available in the medical shop.

Semen once you lost that will not come back – lost is lost.

Effects due to loss of semen – if you not adopt and implement s-formula in your life , you will face lot of problems.

Effects on skull region due to loss of semen – drying, loosening, weakening & falling of hair, mild or severe head ache, pale face with anaemia, eruptions on the face, dark circle around the eye, short slightness, incomplete beard, sunken eyes.

Effects on the trunk region due to loss of semen – pain in shoulder, palpitation of the heart, difficulty in breathing, stomach pain, back pain, gradual degradation of kidneys.

Effects on the genital parts due to loss of semen – wet dreams, incontinence, discharge of semen with urine, premature ejaculation, enlargement of testes, and involuntary urination in sleep.

Effects on the leg region due to loss of semen – pain in thighs, pain in knees, foot pain, palpitation of legs.

Effects on whole body due to loss of semen – wasting of tissues boils on the body, early exhaustion, lack of energy.

Other effects due to loss of semen – physical, mental and moral debility. Mental imbalance, sudden anger, drowsiness, laziness, gloominess, fickle mindedness, lack of thinking power, bad dreams, restlessness of mind, sudden jealousy, sudden fear, lack of muscularity, effeminate or womanish behaviour.

The man who has bad habits, masturbation, wet dreams should give-up the evil habits at once. You will be entirely ruined if you continue the practice. Loss of semen causes your life waste. Yours sex organs, nerves weak, brain failure, heart attack, etc, become weak due to loss of semen. It reduces the lifetime and may die at any time.

Loss of semen makes you loss of health and loss of wealth. Bad characters will born in your mind, mad people increases, peoples behave like devils.

Do not support any activity which causes loss of semen internally or externally in your body.

Loss of semen causes your nerves system weak, brain weak, kidney weak, heart weak, lungs weak, bones weak, sex organs weak. Due to too much loss of semen more diseases will attack, paralysis, piles, mental problems, cruel mind, violence nature. They will give lot of trouble to others, to society, to their family. They spoil the society, spoiling children's, brain will not work properly. Too much wasting of semen will give you idea itself for suicide. Lots of suicide occurs in world due to loss of semen only.

Fever is coming due to lot of wasting of semen in your body. Your body resistance reduces due to loss of semen, due to this reason you will suffer from fever. If you not waste semen, you will never get fever or any type of diseases in your body. Your child also gets fever if you waste lot of semen before marriage. Quality of your child says the quality of your semen.

Quality of your life says the quality of your semen. Quality of your child is fully depending upon the quality of male semen and female semen. Male semen produces sperms and female semen produces ovum.

During the process of reproduction male semen carry sperms to unite with ovum to form zygote. In one ejaculation 20 grams of male semen releases along with sperm. It contains 1% of sperm and 99%

of semen in the volume. Male semen carries all energy from all the parts of your body to create new baby. Male semen is having all the chemical contents, all the properties, all the elements to create new baby. So that it is advised to you use semen only when you need baby. Female semen carry ovum to unite with sperm. Both male semen and female semen combined with sperm and ovum to form zygote. After that zygote will develop by utilizing female semen only. Full development of baby is done by female semen up to nine months. So that it is advised to female do not waste semen, do not pollute semen during pregnancy, follow shastras and sampradayas, and keep distance from your life partner.

When the baby is able to eat food and able to produce semen from food, it will come out of mother stomach. The baby after coming from mother stomach, it starts eating food and start producing semen in body. The body starts growing by using semen. The baby starts developing body and mind fully upto twenty five years. After that semen nourishing, protecting, maintaining body upto seventy five years.

Up to twenty five years all the parts of the body and brain is under developing stage. In this stage, do not waste semen, if you waste semen entire growth of your body stops. Man is incomplete body. This will create lot of problems in your life. It is strictly advised that do not waste single drop of semen throughout your life. But it is allowed once in life time to get child. This is s-formula.

Waste of one drop of semen is the waste of one drop of brain.

If you waste semen, your bones, muscles, tissues, nerves, brain dissolve and converted into liquid and goes out of body through semen. All diseases are coming due to loss of semen only and all the diseases are cured by saving semen in your body.

Following are the reasons which are responsible for semen loss in your body. If you think about sex , masturbation, if you drink alcohol, if you use tobacco, if you eat more salt, more spicy, foods and drinks. If you eat bad food, if you waste salive in your mouth, if you get more sweat, if you waste more tears, if you do more urine, if you talk more, if you hear bad noise, more noise , if you sleep more, if you eat more and more, etc.if you involve all these above said activities, your semen goes out. If you waste more semen, your body grows abnormal.

Failure of digestive system, failure of nerves system, failure of breathing system is due to loss of semen in your body. Entire development of body and mind stops, production of blood stops, development of brain stops, growth of bones stops, production of flesh stops, increasing of fat content, body resistance become low due to loss of semen in your body. Semen is petrol for running all seventy nine organs in our body, it develops controls maitenence of all organs of our body.

Some of the people thinks that semen is present only in male body. We did research on it and come to know that female body is also having semen. All the animals, plants, insects, birds, worms, cells, all living beings inside water, outside water, having semen in their body.

S-formula says that, due to loss of semen only you will suffer gastric and acidity problems. If you waste semen your digestive system becomes very weak and it will not work properly. The acid produced from liver, to digest food, is very strong in nature. To neutralise this acid semen is required. If sufficient semen is not present in your body, you feel burning sensation in your stomach. The entire digestive system is managed and controlled by your semen. If you have already suffering from gastric , acidity problems, you start storing semen in your body, automatically acidity and gastric cured permanently. Keep always the level of semen more than that normal level in your body. So you never get this problem in your life. Medicine is not available for this problem; the only one solution is save semen in your body.

In the same way, cure diabetic disease by saving semen in your body. Semen is insulin to your body. Insulin reduces due to semen loss. Semen maintains insulin level in your body.

High blood pressure and low blood pressure comes only due to loss of semen in your body. Entire nerves system become weak, entire body become weak, blood circulation not goes properly,. There are more than two hundred chemicals present in your body(semen), these chemicals keeps our body normal and healthy. Semen controls blood pressure. Semen controls your blood speed normal and healthy. Due to continues loss of semen speed of blood becomes abnormal. To overcome from this disease save semen in your body. Semen cures blood pressure diseases.

S-formula says that, semen keep the inner body pressure normal level. If you waste semen, your body pressure goes out along with semen. There is no other ways, to go our body pressure ,except through semen. Due to this reason, blood circulation becomes weak, your heart become weak. As pressure decreases, you blood speed decreases, heart will not work properly, you will get heart attack. Cure heart attack diseases by saving semen in your body.in the same way all diseases will attack due to loss of semen only.s-formula says that, if you practice any physical exercises without saving semen, it is very harmful to your health. Any sports, games, dance,karate, yoga, yogasana, gym, wrestling, karate, boxing, etc. Should be practice with saving semen in your body.

Yoga-meaning

21st june, is declared as yoga day. Yoga means save semen, store semen, protect semen in your body. Yoga includes pooja, bhajane, keerthane, prarthane, puranas, punya kathe, dyana, shashtra, sampradaya, dharma palane, bhakthi yoga, karma yoga, hata yoga, raja yoga, dyana yoga, jnana yoga, meditation, pranayama, all cultural programmes related to bhakthi, devine, etc. All must talk on yoga day only the value of semen.

Some people call yogasana in short form yoga, this is wrong concept.

Yoga and yogasana both are different, the benifits are different.

Yoga is a mental exercise and yogasana is a physical exercise.

Yogasana produces semen and yoga save semen.

Yoga+asana=yogasana. One who does yoga must do asana and one who does asana must do yoga. Anybody can do yoga but only healthy person can do yogasana.

Yogasana is a physical exercise, if you do yogasana semen production increases, when the volume of semen increases; your sex organs become strong. Please do not waste semen at this stage. Keep your sex organ always strong. This is the secrete of health.

Yoga is a metal exercise, do yoga only to save semen in your body.

You do any physical exercise only if you are healthy.

The person one who teach yoga, he must a person who saw the god. I am the only one in this world, at present. First you practice yoga, you will get lots of energy, after that you do yogasana or any physical exercises.

A man one who not wasted single drop of semen in his life, he is called healthy man. If he wasted once, he is not healthy man. This is s-formula.

To become perfect human being eat both veg and non veg.

if you eat only veg or only non veg, you body is not in perfect condition. Your body is having some deficiency of nutrients, proteins, enzymes, minerals and energy. You are not a perfect man.

Semen contains more than two hundred chemicals. All these chemicals we are getting only if we eat both veg and nonveg.

Without saving semen in your body, if you worship god, you will not get any benefits from god. Save semen and worship god, you will get whatever you want.

S-formula says that meditation is made for only to save semen in your body. If you store more semen in your body, your body will become highly powerful and highly sensitive. Your panchendriyas, eye, ear, nose, tongue & skin become very sensitive. If you see sex, hear sex, touch anybody, immediately semen goes out. To control your panchendriyas, you must do meditation in good atmosphere around you.

S-formula says that, doctor gives you treatment for diseases; he will not give any treatment to healthy man. Doctor gives good solutions to health problems.

Health teaching is done by your father, mother, teacher, dharma, shahtra, sampradaya etc. Do not spoil your health. The person one who teach about health is need not be a doctor, but the person one who treat diseases must be a doctor. Anybody can teach about health, who knows health secrete.

Yoga guru and doctor, both are opposite words. Yoga guru teaches about health. Doctor gives solutions to problems. Yoga guru is a preventive action, doctor is a corrective action. Prevention is better than cure.

S-formula says that, do not wear skin tight dress, do not expose your body in public places, because people waste more semen and become lazy. Entire society will spoil.

It is very difficult to save semen, store semen and protect semen, but, forcefully we have to control wasting of semen. To save semen or to waste semen, your five sensitive organs are, eyes, ears, nose, tongue and skin are responsible.

Six enemies in your body, kama, krodha, moha, looba, madha and matsara, are born from loss of semen. These enemies become stronger if you waste more semen.

Food will be converted into semen, and then it will be converted into energy. Waste of semen is the waste of energy. Whatever food you eat, it will go out, if you waste semen. Once you waste semen, it is the wastage of food of seventy four days. 20 grams of semen formed from 32 kgs of food.

The person one who waste semen, he will become mad. Due to loss of semen , his brain destroy.

Semen is a pure blood and food for all cells of your body.

Semen is formed from the distillation of blood. Blood filtered seven times to form semen. So that semen is a pure blood.

Sex organs become weak, if you waste semen, sex organs become strong , if you save the semen.

All physical exercises are made for the production of semen and all mental exercises are made to save the semen. Practice all physical exercisesby saving semen, do not practice it by wasting semen. Walking, gym, body building, yogasana, karate, boxing, dance, sports etc. Is very harmfull if you practice by wasting semen.

Semen once you wasted can not be regained. Lost is lost.

If you waste semen, you sleep more and work less , and you will become very lazy. If you save semen, you sleep less and work more, and you always active. If you save semen, naturally you will wake up at 4 o clock, early in the morning.

Waste persons are wasting lot of semen.

Growth of your body becomes abnormal, if you waste semen. Quality of your blood spoils, if you waste semen. Semen always keeps your blood healthy and clean, pure. Semen is a pure blood.

Semen keeps your mind and body in a perfect condition. Your body become delicate, thin, bones visible, no muscular body; your body will not follow mind signals, if you waste semen in your body.

Students become very weak in education, they suffer from loss of memory, due to loss of semen. Body will not follow mind signals if you waste semen.

Fat increase in your body, if you waste more semen. If you save semen, it burns fat and converts fat into body energy. Muscular body comes from saving semen in your body.

You reject marriages, if you waste semen.

Secrete of beauty is hidden semen volume in your body. More semen, more beauty. Less semen, less beauty. Your beauty is your semen. Do not waste semen. White or red, viscous, greasy, oily liquid coming through your sex organs is semen. Do not spoil your beauty.

Do not touch any male in your life. Do not touch any female in your life. If you touch, your semen goes out of your body.

Do not make any activities in front of child, which cause semen loss, if you make it, children's will spoil. If you waste semen, the child born to you will be abnormal and not healthy.

Practice meditation, prnayama, any physical exercises , only when your health is in good condition. Keep always your sex organs strong, if you save semen, your sex organs become very strong.

Semen is your body resistance. It is your body insulin. It cures all diseases. It prevents all diseases attack. Good people never like in semen loss. Semen is having more than two hundred chemicals, proteins, vitamins etc.

Semen is like electrical current in our body. Semen keeps our body, hot in cold region, cold in hot region.

The conservation of semen is very essential to strength of body and mind.

Semen is an organic fluid, seminal fluid.

Look younger, think cleverer, live longer, if you save semen.

The process that results in the discharge of semen is called ejaculation. In one ejaculation of semen will lead to wastage of wealth of energy. Waste of semen is waste of health and wealth.

Angry comes due to wasting of semen, peace of mind comes from saving semen. If you kill semen, it will kill you.

Good people save more semen and bad people waste more semen from their body. Relatives will not help you to waste semen but friends will help you to waste semen. Your father and mother always instruct you indirectly to save semen.mad people becomes good people by saving semen in their body.

Some people save semen without knowing the s-formula concept, they are growing fast, they will become rich in health and wealth. But they do not know that it is because of semen, if you say them the value of semen, they will not believe.

Do not waste semen and do not ejaculate. If you waste you will suffer. Yes it is possible to have multiple orgasms without ejaculating.

Semen is life

Veerya, dhatu, shukra or semen is life. You can attain peace by preserving semen. Its waste means, loss of physical and mental energy. When semen is preserved, it gets reabsorbed by the body and stored in the brain as shakhty or spiritual power. The seminal energy is changed into spiritual energy. This vital force is closely linked with nerves system , so preserve semen to have strong nerves.

The semen is the real vitality n female. Female semen is a hidden treasure in her. It gives a glow to the face, strength to the intellect and wellbeing to the entire body system. Females, to, suffer great loss through having semen loss thoughts and giving way to lust. Vital nerves energy is lost; there is a loss of semen in them as well.

A man's full life span is hundred years or more. This can be achieved only by is a person is save semen. You must have pure character; otherwise, you will lose your vital energy semen. An early death will be the result.

According to psychological and natural laws, the length of human life or any life should be at least five times the period necessary to reach full growth. The horse grows for a period of about three years and lives to be about twelve to fourteen. The camel grows for eight years and lives to be forty. Man grows for about twenty or twenty five years and lives to be about one hundred years or one hundren twenty-five years.

Preservation of semen is no more injurious to the body and soul. The nation of imaginary danger is wasting semen. Virginity is a physical, moral, and intelluctual safe guard to young man. Vital energy is the essence of your body, preservation of it is key to longevity of youthfulness.

Man can live more than thousand years, man can grow up to one hundred feet, only if they save semen.

Evidence of the value of semen for physical & mental health.

Cladius galen of pergamum-<u>claudius galenus</u> of Pergamum (131 - 201ad)

ancient greek physician and philosopher. His works on medicine & philosophy total 22 volumes.

Hippocrates and galen believed that semen came from all humors of the body.

Involuntary loss was termed 'gonorrhoea': 'it robs the body of its vital breath'; 'losing sperm amounts to losing the vital spirits'; exhaustion, weakness, dryness of the whole body, thinness, eyes growing hollow, are the resulting symptoms.

Aristotle-Aristotle (350bc)

if you haven't heard of him you have learnt too much in sex-ed.

If men start to engage in sexual activity at too early an age... This will affect the growth of their bodies.

Nourishment that would otherwise make the body grow is diverted to the production of semen. ... Aristotle is saying that at this stage the body is still growing; it is best for sexual activity to begin when its growth is 'no longer abundant', for when the body is more or less at full height, the transformation of nourishment into semen does not drain the body of needed material.

For aristotle, semen is the residue derived from nourishment, that is of blood, that has been highly concocted to the optimum temperature and substance. This can only be emitted by the male as only the male, by nature of his very being, has the requisite heat to concoct blood into semen.

'sperms are the excretion of our food, or to put it more clearly, as the most perfect component of our food'.

Democritus- democritus **(400 bc) of abdera thrace was called "the laughing philosopher"**
how he could be so happy without having a date

with rosy palm and her five daughters is beyond me (and beyond modern medicine too).

"coition", said democritus, "is a kind of epilepsy." "it is", said haller, "an action very similar to a convulsion, and which of itself astonishingly weakens and affects the whole nervous system."

"democritus, an ancient physician, believed that this semen was derived from the whole body "particularly the important parts such as bones, flesh and sinews."

Pythagoras -of the pythagorean theorem fame. If he was smart enough to figure out a triangle you can be sure he could figure out how to go for a few days without jerking his gerkin.

Pythagoras advocated continence as a practice of utmost physiological value both to body and brain, for he considered the semen as 'the flower of the purest blood,'

Pythagoras taught that there was a direct connection between the semen and the brain and that loss of semen weakens the brain, while its conservation improves brain's nutrition, since the substances thus conserved act as brain nutrients.

Dr.Paulcharlesdubois (1848-1918)
siwss neurologist, professor, writer and pioneer of psychotherapy

Ssexual indulgence, not continence, is the cause of neurasthenia

Agustehenriforel (1848-1931)
swiss myrmecologist, neuroanatomist and psychiatrist, notable for his investigations into the brain structure of humans and ant.

"abstinence, or sexual continence, is by no means impractical for a normal young man of average constitution, assiduous in intellectual and physical work and abstaining from artificial excitants", adding, "the idea is current among young people that abstinence is something abnormal and impossible, and yet the many who observe it prove that chastity can be practiced without prejudice to health".

Dr.Jeanalfredfournier(1832-1914)
french dermatologist, professor and medical writer,

Professor alfred fournier, a physiologist of note, ridicules the idea of "the dangers of continence for the young man", and that during his years of medical practice, he has never come across one such case.

Dr. Charles marie edouard chassaignac
french surgical pioneer,

Chassaignac claims that the healthier the individual, the easier to practice complete abstinence; it is only the diseased and neurotic person who finds it difficult to do so.

Professor charles edouard brown sequard

(1817 - 1894)

british physiologist and neurologist

brown-sequard has shown that spermatic secretions increase nerve and brain vitality.[1]

Brown sequard discovered that the voluntary supression of the ejaculation of semen strengthens a man and is conducive to long life. This is due to the semen being thus returned to the body which thus acts as a tonic for the nervous system.

Dr.Oskar,lassar
German dermatologist

Sexual continence is not injurious to young men.

Dr. William acton (1813 - 1875)
british doctor and medical writer.
Authored functions and disorders of the
reproductive organs in childhood, youth, adult

age, and advanced life considered in their physiological, social, and moral relations. (1894)

Chastity no more injures the body than the soul

Acton says that "it is only mature individuals who can bear even infrequent acts of copulation without more or less injury. In young persons all the vital powers should be conserved for growth and development.

In a state of health no sexual impression should ever affect a child's mind or body. All its vital energy should be employed in building up the growing frame, in storing up external impressions, and educating the brain to receive them.

Dr. Claude-francois lalleman
french surgeon, (1790 - 1853)

Lallemand warned that loss of sperm could be dangerous to health.

Lalleman traces spermatorrhea to an inflammation, congestion and hypersecretion of the mucous membranes of the urethra, primarily initiated by frequent sexual orgasms and intensified by the irritation of toxic blood resulting from wrong diet and autointoxication. Alcohol, coffee, tea and spices, by irritating the genital mucous membranes, he believes to contribute to this condition.

Dr. Leopold deslandes md (1796 - 1850) french medical writer and doctor. Member of the royal academy of medicine, paris

Deslandes observes: "the diseases affecting the nervous system, that system which is powerfully disturbed by coition, are not the only ones resulting from venereal excess. We shall see that all alterations of tissue, every physical disorder, may be caused by this. We may fearlessly assert that most of the inconveniences and diseases afflicting the human species arise from venereal excesses."

Dr. Simon-auguste-andre-david tissot (1728-1787) swiss professor of medicine

He followed in the tradition of the greek medicine when he wrote that the body is an energy system which needs constant care to maintain equilibrium.[1]

'losing one ounce of sperm is more debilitating than losing forty ounces of blood', in treatise on the diseases produced by onanism.his tenet was that debility, disease and death are the outcome of semen loss

Tissot describes as follows the effects of sexual excess:

"the debility caused by these excesses derange the functions of all organs... Digestion, perspiration and evacuation do not take place in their usual healthy manner; ... And astonishing weakness in the back, debility of the genital organs, bloody urine, deranged appetite, headache and numerous other diseases ensue; in a word, nothing shortens life so much as the abuse of sexual pleasures... Excesses in the gratification of sexual desire not only cause the diseases of languor, but sometimes acute diseases; and they always produce irregularities in those affections which depend on other causes, and very readily render them malignant when the energies of nature are at fault."

Dr. Arnold lorand
austrian doctor and author

The ancient hindoos recommended to men sexual abstinence of long duration, thinking that by this means the internal secretion of the sexual glands would be absorbed into the system and that they would thereby reap all the benefits inherent in such a secretion. By this it seems that thousands of years before claude bernard and brown-sequard the hindoos already appreciated the great importance of the internal secretions.

Dr. Leopold lowenfeld (1857 - 1924)
german gynecologist, psychiatrist and author

The gynecologist, loewenfeld, considers it possible for a sexually normal individual to live in permanent continence without any ill-effects whatsoever.

Dr. Herbert macgolfin shelton (1895 - 1985), **natural hygienist.**

By producing enervation and by exciting the nervous system, dr. Shelton claims that sexual excess can further the development of any disease to which the individual is subject.

"no function is so exhausting to the whole system as this. If excessively indulged in, no practice can possibly be so enervating.

"what constitutes excess? The reply has been given: anything is excess when procreation is not the end. Man is sexually perverted. He is the only animal that has his `social problem,' the only animal that supports prostitution, the only animal that practices self-abuse, the only animal that is demoralized by all forms of sexual perversions, the only animal whose male will attack the females, the only animal where the desire of the female is not the law, the only one that does not exercise his sexual powers in harmony with their primitive constitution."

Dr. Rita sapiro finkler (1888 - 1968)
pioneer endocrinologist, founded the department of endocrinology a the beth israel hospital.

Finkler answered that sexual continence is not injurious to young men, but, on the contrary, is beneficial to body and mind.

Arthur hiler ruggles
president of the american psychiatric association

Ruggles writes: "sexual abstinence is compatible with perfect health and tends to increase vitality through resorption of the semen."

Max thorek (1880 - 1960)
surgeon, writer and professor of medicine & plastic surgery

The gonad elaborates through its internal secretions the chemical products which are taken up by the circulation and carried to the central nervous system, and there erotization results. That these substances of internal secretion have a selective action seems probable, and that such substances are stored in the central nervous system, seems, in view of recent experiments, quite certain... O'malleey thinks that the direct action of the chemical products of the gonads through the nervous system influences the growth and increased metabolism of every tissue of the body. That there is a direct relationship between the gonads and the hypophysis is fairly well established... Since the time of hippocrates and aristotle, it has been believed that there was a coordination between the testicular fluid and the nervous system, brain and cord."

<u>Sir robert mccarrison</u> (1878 - 1960) british physician to the king (1928 - 1935), knighted for his medical work

Mccarrison, found that atrophy of the testicles is frequently found in cerebral and spinal diseases.

Francis hugh adam marshall (1878 - 1949) eminent english physiologist at edinburgh university

Marshall, in his "introduction to sex physiology", points out the need for such restraint over the reproductive function and the sublimation of sex energy into higher cerebral forms of expression, as was the case with many intellectual geniuses of the past, who led continent lives.

Sir frederick walker mott (1853 - 1926) neurologist, author and pioneer of british biochemistry.

Tthe majority of these insane subjects studied by mott were habitual masturbators, which practice should have a relation to their testicular degeneration, which mott considers the primary cause of their brain involution and degeneration. Mott's observations were confirmed by obregia, parhon and urechia . Who also found degeneration of the seminiferous tubules and absence of spermatogenesis in dementia praecox. These investigators conclude that spermatozoa may have an internal function that is necessary for the normal metabolism of the brain, and that dementia praecox may be due to an alteration or deficiency of their production due to degeneration of the seminiferous tubules of auto-intoxication.

Mohandas k. Gandhi

'The horror with which ancient literature regarded the fruitless loss of the vital fluid was not a superstition born of ignorance. . . Surely it is criminal for a man to allow his most precious possession to run to wasle.'

Talk with margaret sanger, 1935, dr. Bernard. R.w., nutritional sex control & rejuvenation. Health research: pomeroy.

Dr. Dr s chidambaranathan, homeopathic doctor

Semen is a rich source of calcium, phosphorus, lecithin, cholesterol, nucleoproteins, iron, vitamin-e, sodium, magnesium, etc. So, excessive loss of semen will deprive our body of calcium, phosphorus, lecithin, etc. Researchers find many similarities between cerebrospinal fluid (which nourishes the brain and nervous system) and semen in constituents/composition.

<u>Dr. Charles eucharist de medicis sajous</u> (1852 - 1929)
physician, endocinologist, teacher, author, and editor.

Sajous states his conviction that the myelin of the nerves is not a mere insulating material or sheath, but a phosphorus-containing substance (lecithin) which, when in contact with oxygen-laden blood, generates nerve-electricity through oxidation. The importance of sufficient lecithin to keep the myelin sheaths properly nourished is therefore apparent. ... The lecithin and lipins of the myelin sheaths have a nutritive function in relation to the nerves. ... "lecithin, therefore, becomes the functional ground-substance of the cell- body of the neuron, just as it is in the nerve. Both in the neuron and its continuation, the nerve, therefore, the vascular fibrils carry blood-plasma, which, by passing through their walls, maintains a continuous reaction, of which the phosphorus of the lecithin and the oxygen of the blood-plasma are main reagents, and chemical energy is the end-result."

Dr. Edward charles spitzka (1852 - 1914)
brain anatomist, neurologist, and psychiatrist

Excessive venery and masturbation have from time immemorial been supposed to be the direct causes of insanity. Unquestionably they exert a deleterious influence on the nervous system, and may provoke insanity partly through their direct influence on the nervous centres, partly through their weakening effect on the general nutrition. That there is a close connection between pathological nervous states and the sexual function is exemplified in the satyriasis of mania and the early stages of paretic dementia as well as in the sexual delusion of monomania and the abnormal genital sensations of that condition.

In his "masturbatic insanity," dr. Spitzka presents a study of twelve cases of insanity, all of which he attributes to masturbation. He claims that the occurrence of psychoses as the result of masturbation is primarily due to arrested brain nutrition. This results from the withdrawal from the circulation of brain-nourishing lecithin and other phosphorus compounds through excessive seminal discharges. For we must remember that lecithin is a chief constituent of the myelin sheaths of nerve-cells and essential for their activity, during which it is consumed--for it is the nerve-oil that keeps the fire of nerve and brain activity burning. Since lecithin is also a principal constituent of the semen, we can readily understand why excessive sexual activity should lead to lecithin deficiency and undernutrition of nerve and brain cells.

Max von gruber (1853 - 1927) austrian physician, bacteriologist, and hygienist.

It is absurd to regard the semen as an injurious secretion like the urine, which requires periodic evacuation, but as vital fluid which is not only reabsorbed during sexual abstention, but this reabsorption appears to have a beneficial effect on the physiological economy, as shown by the large number of intellectual geniuses who have led continent lives.

Frequent discharges of semen lead to a "reduction of the peculiar internal secretion of the testes," which is otherwise resorbed into the blood-stream. The immediate effects of sexual excess, he states, are depression, fatigue and exhaustion. As further symptoms there is pressure in the lumbar region, nervous irritability, a feeling of pressure in the head, stupidity, insomnia, ringing in the ears, spots before the eyes, shunning of light, a feeble trembling and actual shaking, pounding of the heart, tendency to sweating and muscular weakness. There is also weakness of memory, neurasthenia, melancholic depression and disinclination to physical or mental effort. The digestive activity becomes less efficient and food is less well utilized. There is a deficiency in blood and a lowered resistance to infectious bacteria, the tubercle bacillus in particular, for which reason sexual excess is known to predispose to consumption aside from its tendency to drain the body of calcium. There is irritable weakness of the genitals, premature ejaculation, frequent nocturnal emissions, and increasing impotence. The more frequent nocturnal emissions that result increase the nervous irritability and exhaustion (i.e., neurasthenia). All these effects are more marked in the young and the aged; in the former, sexual excess, by its detrimental influence on metabolism and the process of growth, stunts physical and mental development, while in the aged it hastens death, often by causing heart failure.

G. Frank lydston (1858 - 1923)

professor of genito-urinary surgery and syphilology in the medical departmentof the university of illinois ; professor of surgery, chicago clinical chool, chicago, illinois.

"continence per se, probably never is harmful. The non- elimination of the seminal secretion from the testes often is productive of great bodily and mental vigor." in his opinion, "one may be perfectly healthy and physically vigorous while leading a life of absolute continence."

Professor lydston mentions cases of apoplexy, paralysis and fatal cardiac conditions occurring in predisposed persons as the result of sexual excess. "from a priori considerations," he writes, "involving the immediate effects of sexual excitement and indulgence upon the brain and spinal cord, we might naturally expect insanity to be a frequent result of masturbation and excessive venery." while the majority of persons are protected against such serious affects upon the cerebrospinal functions by their natural resistance, in those in whom this resistance nervous equilibrium incidental to faulty or imperfect nerve structure, whether due to heredity, congenital defect or acquired disease, the conditions are different. Under such circumstances, repeated sexual orgasms, according to prof. Lydston, can procure "actual structural alterations of nerve-fibers and cells and vessals of the brain, with coincident psychopathic phenomena," which "are naturally to be expected as occasional results of these severe and repeated shocks to the susceptible nervous system produced by the sexual orgasms."

According to prof. Lydston, the results of sexual excess are similar to those of masturbation, and both result from the disturbance of blood chemistry and general metabolism caused by the withdrawal from the body of the substances of which the semen is composed: calcium, phosphorus, lecithin, cholesterol, albumen, iron, etc. Though physical impairment, as well as mental impairment, from sexual excess is very common, less attention, has been paid to it than to the evil results of masturbation, in view of the current belief that, unlike masturbation, coitus is harmless under all circumstances. However it is lydston's opinion that "sexual excess is the most prolific cause of that most civilized and most fashionable of all hydra-headed diseases, neurasthenia, adding, "moderation in sexual intercourse is not only conducive to prolonged virility, but to longevity. It is certain that many cases of neurasthenia in both male and female are due to sexual excess."

In an article, "sexual neurasthenia and the prostate" (medical record, feb., 1912), prof. F. G. Lydston presents evidence to prove that neurasthenia has its roots in prostatic dysfunction caused by sexual indulgence, which results in depletion and derangement of the prostatic hormone. He writes: "there is almost always some functional derangement of the sexual apparatus behind which lies a varying degree of organic disorder (in neurasthenia). My experience leads me to the conclusion that neurasthenia in the males is associated with prostatic hyperemia and hyperesthesis of the prostatic urethra more than with any other condition.... Practically all of these subjects have been masturbators, many of them have indulged in sexual excesses, and not a few have had gonorrhea.... I doubt if it is possible for one to indulge in either masturbation or sexual excess for any length of time without producing disturbance of prostatic circulation and innervation... Practically every masturbator who has practiced the habit for any length of time may be considered as having a more or less tender and swollen prostate. My experience goes to show that this condition underlies many of the cases of nocturnal emissions with which we meet."

"as might be inferred from the fact that sexual excess and masturbation bear an important relation to locomotor ataxia, spermatorrhea is associated with that form of nervous disease more often than any other. The evil habit of masturbation, if continued, produces great irritation of the procreative organs -- especially of the seat of sexual sensibility in the prostatic urethra... Erotic dreams result, with losses of seminal secretion. This may merge into true spermatorrhea, the morbid condition finally becoming so pronounced that with little or no provocation, losses occur in the daytime. "spermatorrhea, in the majority of instances is the result of sexual excess or masturbation, and, moreover, the effects of the venereal organs being expended upon the nervous system, it is rational to infer that the disease when fully developed essentially is a neurosis."

Dr. Frederick humphreys md **(1816 - 1900)** homeopathic doctor and founder of the new york state homeopathic medical society. Writer of "manual of homeopathic remedies (1930) and many other works.

Nervous debility is often brought on in young person's by the habit of masturbation, which, if persisted in from time to time, is inevitably followed by consequences immediate and remote, and are of the most formidable character.[1]

"[nervous debility] is almost invariably the result of some drain upon the vital forces, such as excesses of various kinds: excessive morbid indulgence, involuntary losses of vital fluids, too long and too constant excitement of the sexual system, and more especially when such indulgences are allowed in connection with mental and physical overwork. Nervous debility is often brought on in young person's by the habit of masturbation, which, if persisted in from time to time, is inevitably followed by consequences immediate and remote, and are of the most formidable character.

Dr. Oskar lassar
german dermatologist

Sexual continence is not injurious to young men.

Professor charles edouard brown sequard

(1817 - 1894)

british physiologist and neurologist

brown-sequard has shown that spermatic secretions increase nerve and brain vitality.

Brown sequard discovered that the voluntary supression of the ejaculation of semen strengthens a man and is conducive to long life. This is due to the semen being thus returned to the body which thus acts as a tonic for the nervous system.

Dr. Leopold casper (1859-1959)
highly regarded berlin urologist. Founder of ureteral catheterisation and functional renal diagnostics.

The nervous system's power of resistance, especially that of the affected centers, is so slight that the most trivial stimulation produces the maximum of irritability, as the result of which ejaculation ensues; or, conversely, the normal tonicity of the ejaculatory duct is raised to the highest point, so that the semen flows away spontaneously or escapes upon the slightest pressure.

Thus, sexual excesses may cause this symptom, either directly or by inducing neurasthenia. Of the sexual excesses masturbation occupies the first rank; it is immaterial whether it be physical, that is, practised by frictioning the penis, or only psychical, an ejaculation being induced by conjuring up voluptuous fancies.

At present we do not believe in the dreadful results of masturbation described by lallemand and tissot, but yet it must be conceded that if the habit is persisted in for years it will impair the soundness of both body and mind, that it will result in enfecblement and hyperaesthesia of the nervous system. It is not so much the numerous losses of semen as it is the effect of the frequently repeated stimulation upon the nervous system which brings about this condition. The frequency with which masturbation is practised explains why abnormal pollutions result more frequently from this habit than from sexual excesses.

Casper regarded spermatorrhea [the involuntary emission of semen without orgasm] and neurasthenia [nervous disorders] as going hand in hand, and that both result from excessive seminal losses through sexual excess.

Dr. George miller beard **(1839 - 1883)**
**yale graduate who went on to become a
distinguished doctor, medical writer and
researcher.**

Dr. Beard notes that [american] indian boys do not masturbate and young men remain chaste until marriage, conditions which we do not find among so-called civilized races.[1]

Neurasthenia has a sexual origin, the weakened condition of the nerves being intimately related to the sexual life of the individual. He came to the conclusion that neurasthenia has its origin in abnormal functioning of the sexual organs by the observation that in patients who came to him with functional nervous diseases, examination invariably showed that there was a condition of inflammation of the prostatic urethra. He wrote: "in men, as in women, a large group of nervous symptoms, which are very common indeed, would not exist but for morbid states in the reproductive system... A morbid state of this part of the body is both an effect and a cause of nervous exhaustion."

Beard then proceeded to determine what caused this morbid condition in the reproductive organs (inflammation of the prostatic urethra), which he considered the predisposing cause of neurasthenia. A study of the symtomatology of spermatorrhea, a disease characterized by an involuntary loss of sexual secretions (in the urine, after defecation, or at other times), led him to a solution of this problem. Beard noted that spermatorrhea was a frequent symptom of all kinds of neurasthenic as well as other debilitating diseases, and that there was a direct relationship between the amount of seminal fluid discharged and the intensity of the nervous symptoms. He also found that frequent nocturnal emissions likewise led to neurasthenic symptoms.

"scminal emissions," he concluded, are frequently the cause of nervous and other diseases." in spite of their universality (among civilized males, but not among animals), beard believed that nocturnal emissions are pathological; and like spermatorrhea, a related condition of seminal emission, they are suscepstantially cured, he stated. This, he claimed, by the conservation of nerve- nourishing seminal constituents that results, would markedly reduce the nervous symptoms thus produced.

As the result of his observations, beard came to the conclusion that neurasthenia is a direct effect of the withdrawal from the blood of certain chemical substances needed for the nutrition of nervous tissue, which results from seminal discharges; and that the loss of considerable quantities of seminal fluid, involuntarily or voluntarily, leads to undernourishment of the cells of the central nervous system, causing them to be weakened and exhausted. He also pointed out that this condition is usually associated with an inflammatory state of the prostatic urethra "which is so often the source whence all these difficulties originate, and by which they are maintained." the prostatic urethra, he claimed, is the most important center of reflex irritation of the body, a morbid state of which is both an effect and cause of nervous exhaustion.

Dr. Joseph william howe **(1843 - 1890) professor of clinical surgery at bellevue hospital medical school**

Dr. Howe, professor of clinical surgery at bellevue hospital medical school, believes that sclerosis of nerve fibers of the cerebellum may be caused by involuntary emissions of semen by night or day. He also thinks that "diseases of the brain and cord are ushered in and accompanied by frequent ejaculations of seminal fluid. Many of the cases are accompanied by impotence, others develop satyriasis and priapism. He adds:

"in one case of partial cerebral sclerosis which involved a small portion of the cerebellum, the patient suffered from frequent emissions before any symptoms of cerebral trouble manifested themselves. Coincident with manifestations of the sclerosis, the pollutions were increased in frequency, and as the disease progressed, were of daily and nightly occurrence.

"progressive locomotor ataxia was at one time supposed to arise from inordinate sexual congress and onanism.... A majority of patients suffering from locomotor ataxia have spermatorrhea of troublesome nature. In the later stages of the disease there is complete loss of virile power. In the cases which are preceded by spermatorrhea, the disease is of a more serious nature, and is more apt to run a rapid course and reach a fatal termination.

"other diseases of the spinal cord, such as white softening, tumors and injuries, are all accompanied by some disarrangement of the genital functions. In some instances, they are characterized by frequent ejaculations and loss of virility; in others priapism and aspermitism are present. In injuries which produce a certain amount of irritation and inflammation, the latter conditions are more likely to be present, while in anemic conditions, or chronic softening, seminal emissions and impotence are usual. Chronic or white softening of the spinal cord may arise as a result of masturbation and sexual excess."

Dr. Charles arthur mercier (1852 - 1919)
english psychiatrist and author of several books on neuroscience

With each reproductive act the bodily energy is diminished; the capacity for exertion is lessened; the languor and lassitude that follow indicate the strain that has been put upon the forces of the body, the amount of energy that has been abstracted from the store at the disposal of the organism.

Now, the seat of the reservoir of energy is the nervous system, and any drain upon the energies of the body is a drain on the nervous system, whose highest regions will, on the general grounds already familiar, be the first and most affected. Hence the reproductive act has an effect on the highest regions of the nervous system which is of the nature of a stress, and tends to produce disorder. With a normally constituted organism the stress of the reproductive act is not sufficient to produce disorder, unless it is repeated with undue frequency ; on the contrary, by providing a natural and legitimate outlet for surplus activity, its influence is distinctly beneficial. But in an organism whose energies are naturally defective, the tendency of the reproductive act will be to increase the deficiency ; and in an organism which is inherently below the normal stability, the tendency of the stress of the reproductive act will be to produce disorder.

This tendency will be especially severe when indulgence in the sexual act is begun at too early an age.

Hence it is in males chiefly that are exhibited the ill-consequences of excessive sexual indulgence ; and in the male sex a very large proportion of cases of dementia are either due to, or are aggravated, enhanced, and prolonged, by undue sexual indulgence.

There are an enormous number of cases, forming together a considerable proportion of the total population, in which premature decadence of the mental powers, premature exhaustion of the energies, premature inability for vigorous and active exertion, result from excessive sexual indulgence in early life. The young man, full of vigour, boiling over, as it were, with energy and activity, recently let loose from the restraint of school or college, unaccustomed to control himself or to deny himself any gratification, launches out into excesses which at the time appear to be indulged in with impunity. But sooner or later comes the day of reckoning. He has felt himself possessed of abundance of energy, and he has dissipated it lavishly, feeling that after each wasteful expenditure he had more to draw upon ; but he is in the position of a spendthrift who is living on his capital. Had he husbanded his resources and lived with moderation, the interest on his capital would have sufficed to keep him in comfort to old age ; but he has lavished his capital, has lived a few short years in great profusion, and before middle life he is a beggar.

Hippocrates- you remember hearing about the hippocratic oath, right? So why this "father of medicine" didn't approve of greasing your monkey everyday to fall asleep is beyond the scope of modern medicine. We are after all, "advanced."

Hippocrates and galen believed that semen came from all humors of the body.

Since the time of hippocrates and aristotle, it has been believed that there was a coordination between the testicular fluid and the nervous system, brain and cord.

The ancients note a relation between the semen and the spinal cord, and hippocrates believed that involuntary seminal losses can cause tabes dorsalis. That they cause spinal weakness is well known.

Hippocrates called the disease *tabes dorsalis*. He says "it proceeds from the spinal cord, and is frequently met with among newly married people and libertines. There is no fever, the appetite is preserved, but the body falls away. If you interrogate the patients, they will tell you that they feel as if ants were crawling down the spine. If they have connection the congress is fruitless;they lose semen in bed, whether they are troubled with lascivious dreams or not. They lose on horseback or in walking. Their breathing becomes difficult; they fall into a state of feebleness, and suffer from a weight in the head and a singing in the ears. If in this condition, they become affected with a strong fever, and die with cold extremities.

Traditional

This theory that semen comes from the body is an ayurvedic understanding wherein different materials of the body "distill" to form purer substances which are then extracted by the testicles as semen. The fact that semen comes from the testicles is no big discovery. The value of semen was stressed by ancient philosophers & doctors.

The basic principles of ayurveda involve a metaphysical understanding of the elements. The bodies tissues are divided into seven:

Rasa (plasma),Rakta (blood),Mamsa (muscle),Meda (fat tissues),Asthi (bone),Majja (marrow),Shukra (semen)

The semen can be extracted by the testicles or reabsorbed to strengthen the body and brain.

Semen is a mysterious secretion that is able to create a living body. Semen itself is living substance. It is life itself. Therefore, when it leaves man, it takes a portion of his own life. A living thing cannot be put to laboratory tests, without first killing it. The scientist has no apparatus to test it. God has provided the only test to prove its precious nature, viz., the womb. The very fact that semen is able to create life is proof enough that it is life itself.

I have thousands of letters from young men who have wasted this precious fluid and are in a miserable plight. Several young men even go to the point of committing suicide! Through reckless waste of semen, they lose all their physical, mental and intellectual faculties. Those who are perfect brahmacharins have lustrous eyes, a healthy body and mind, and a keen, piercing intellect.

Scientists with their test tubes and balances cannot approach subtle things. No amount of dissection of the body will be able to tell you where the soul is, where life is, or where the mind is. Through the practice of yoga, the seminal energy— not the gross physical semen— flows upwards and enriches the mind. This has been declared by the sages. You will have to experience it yourself.

-- swami shivananda

Semen is the most powerful energy in the world.

Semen is great, He does good things and everything He does is for a reason, Yes He is real, He is in my heart. I once met the richest man on Earth. He was a begger who slept under a bridge. But he had Semen. Semen is always with you… You just need to pay attention.

The poorest man on earth who is friends with semen is richer than the richest man who is not friends with semen, "Only Semen can Judge Me?" People can and will Judge me everyday but Semen will only judge me ONCE and His judgment is the

ONLY one that matters."Semen is not my "co- pilot", he is in full control.Who are you to judge? Leave the jugding to Semen, he who judges others will be judged.

When your life is beginning to turn bad, when things arent going your way, when all around you begins to fade, Semen plan for you becomes bigger and better than before. He lives in me, and im only 16. Let him live, and share through you.

I don't know who wrote half of these... But that is really messed up! Semen is real. I don't know who you are or what you are thinking... But I know he lives in me each and every day and no matter what happeneds I will still love him!

Be kind to other even if they are not to you, Keep spreading love even if you don't get it back, Be helpful even if you have no one to help you, Do not change yourself according to others, Just remember one thing it is not between you and others it is always between you and the Semen.

Semen is real and he is living in me! .He is the only light in this world. I believe in the SUN even when it isn't shining, I believe in LOVE even when I don't feel it, and I believe in SEMEN even when he is silent. Don't tell your Semen how big your storm is, tell your storm how big your Semen is....
Semen is great. He does good things and everything He does is for a reason.Yes He is real!! He is in my heart.

I once met the richest man on Earth. He was a begger who slept under a bridge. But he had Semen.Semen is always with you… You just need to pay attention. The poorest man on earth who is friends with semen is richer than the richest man who is not friends with semen,When we pray, Semen hears more than we say, answers more than we ask, gives more than we imagine, in his own time and in his own way.

Dear Semen, if one day I lose my hope and purpose, give me confidence that your destiny is better than anything I ever dreamed. You may feel lost and alone, but Semen knows exactly where you are, and He has a good plan for your life. Semen is love and I love Semen…he can't break my heart. Semen's "no" is not a rejection, it's a redirection.

When the toughest of the problems strike me, I just remind myself that Semen is on my side.

Semen, if I can't have what I want, let me want what I have. You can hate me, or you can love me, but in the end, only SEMEN can judge me. Atheists have one reason for not beliving in Semen, it's called "Fear". Yet those who believe in Semen have no Fear, for their Semen is with them and there wasn't, isn't and won't be anything to Fear as long as he's there.

Semen is the one who lives in me. i love him with all of my heart i want to be a light that when people look at me they see semen inside of me. The people who don't believe you will really regrete when he comes back and you will reqalize that he is real and you had wished that you did it right from the beginning i love him and I know for a fact he loves me .

Many people turn to Semen when life has them down but forget to keep in touch with him when he turns it all around. Semen is like the universe you can't see it but can believe it , Semen, sometimes takes us into troubled waters, not to drown us but to cleanse us.The poorest man in the world is not the one who doesn't have a single cent but the one who doesn't have SEMEN.

When his life was ruined, his family killed, his farm destroyed, Job knelt down on the ground and yelled up to the heavens, "Why semen? Why me?" and the thundering voice of Semen answered, There's just something about you that pisses me off.

Semen can turn water into wine, but he can't turn your whining into anything. semen grace is bigger than your sins. I asked for strength… And Semen gave me difficulties to make me strong. I asked for wisdom… And Semen gave me problems to solve. I asked for prosperity… And Semen gave me a brain and energy to work. I asked for courage… And Semen gave me danger to overcome. I asked for love… And Semen gave me troubled people to help. I asked for favors… And Semen gave me opportunities. I recieved nothing I wanted, But I received everything I needed.

Religion may be the cause of war. RELIGION, not Semen! Man is the cause of war. If man would take the time to listen to each other rather then dive head first into the ice cold water, if they would just analyze the situation many men, women and children would still be here today. So maybe Religion is the cause of war, but only the misunderstanding of religion cause war. NOT SEMEN.

Semen always listen to your prayer… Only we have to be patient for the answer. Sometimes Semen doesn't change your situation because He's trying to change your heart. Don't forget to pray today, because Semen didn't forget to wake you up this morning. "Semen gives the sweets to the man with no teeth"

Semen doesn't give you what you want… He creates the opportunity for us to do so.

Don't give up. Semen will give you the strength you need to hold on.He who says I m alone…had never listened to SEMEN who is always with him. Semen is the alpha and omega, The beginning and the end, Cast all your cares on Him and He will guide you through all your troubles and worries, just ask Him…Its Easy. Semen is good, all the times.

Semen put you in this world not so you could please the likes of others but so you can live your life to the fullest and please Him and Him only! Semen is everywhere- no one has actually experienced living without Him… He's everywhere, even if you don't believe.

Semen works in mysterious way!!! Don't get mad when you cannot achieve what you want… there is a right time semen will give you… and believe in your heart…

Rules to a better life 1. Never Hate 2. Don't worry 3. Live simply 4. Expect a little 5. Give a lot 6. Always smile 7. Live with love. 8. Best of all, Be with Semen 101 When Semen gives us a "No" for an answer, keep in mind that there is a much greater "Yes" behind it. His "No" is not a "Rejection" but a "Redirection."

Throughout life people will make you mad, disrespect you and treat you bad. Let Semen deal with things they do, cause hate in your heart will consume you too. Friends will let down, but Semen will never let down. Semen is merciful.

I'm 13 years old and I've need Semen every second that I breathe. Every day that I continue living is another day I have to thank him for letting me. Don't think of Semen as a just a friend, he is someone to try to impress, yes he will love you through it all but that doesn't mean you shouldn't try your hardest to do your best. He will lead you through anything you need, if it's ruff at times always remember everything happens for a reason. "If he got you to it, you can get yourself through it."

Semen is stronger than my circumstances.Semen is our refuge and strength. A very present help in trouble, therefore we will not fear.Semen is my Strength and my refuge. Semen is everywhere. A real human doesn't use Semen name for his bad intentions to others. "You know if you want Semen to speak to you; you must speak to Semen."

I will lift up my voice and praise you always. You are the Alpha and Omega, S-formula of s-formulas and the love of my life. I will be praying for all that deny you.

If you don't believe your almighty Saviour, just look out the window!! How could something so beautiful and complex be there by chance!? If can't!! And how could man be descendants of apes or other animals, when humans are so mysterious and animals so simple? Do animals feel emotionally? No. They may be attached to their owner, but they don't feel pain, compassion, love, joy, anger, and other such strong emotions!! Humans could only have been made from a Creator that knew what He was doing. And yes, Semen created both man and woman in His image. That means we both have characteristics of Semen. Semen is like a man and a woman, or they are like Him at least, but He is also much greater! If we understood Semen completely, what fulfillment would that bring us? Would we still want to seek Him if there was nothing left to seek? No. Because Semen wants us to seek Him, and in time he will reveal Himself in different ways to co- inside with your life. All you need is a little faith.

Semen is the best thing that has ever happened to me. I am only 14 and I accepted energy into my heart when I was 6. My life has some complications in it and I have often wondered where Semen was. I look back and I realize that while I was hurting and crying out to Semen, he was right there beside me holding my hand and helping me get through it. He was hurting because I was in pain. He loves me more that I can imagine! I look outside and I see his majesty in everything, the little details in the butterfly's wing, in all the different kinds of flowers, in the sunrises and sunsets. When I lie in bed during a thunderstorm it reminds me of His amazing power. Semen has done many things for me and he has comforted me when no one else could.

Before Semen we are all equally wise and equally foolish. Semen is like the wind. We can't see him, but we know He's there. Be high with SEMEN, not with DRUGS. Faith in Semen is the best medicine…

Semen Answers ALL peoples; It's just that sometimes his Answers Aren't what you want. The secret of true happiness is trusting in Semen. The sun, the moon, the stars, the birds, the animals, the flowers, are all proof that a universal power exists.

I don't care what others think the only person im trying my hardest to impress is the big man upstairs named SEMEN! Semen always gives us a red signal whenever we are about to make a mistake, but it's our selfish mind and ego which never understands his signals which sometimes leads to incidents or accidents.

I have amazing potential. I can make good choices. I am never alone. I can do hard things. I am beautiful inside and out. I am of great worth. He has a plan for me. I know who I am. A daughter of Semen. Trust semen and he will lead you to the right direction…I believe in Semen because he believes in me. Trust in him, believe in him, and love him, and good things will happen. He loves you and when things get tough, know he is always there. Even when you don't feel him around you, he is always there. Tonight I turn all my worries over to Semen. He will be up all night anyway.

Smile. Just smile. Smile at those who don't have Him in their hearts. Go ahead. Smile. And while you are at it, try to tell them about Him. And keep on smiling when they push you away and tell you that He isn't real and that there is no proof that He exists. And then when you just can't smile any wider, laugh. Laugh till it hurts then finally ask them: "Do you have any proof that He doesn't?" And you don't have to say another word even if they do. Cause you won. YOU WON. Cause having proof that Semen is real totally ruins the point in believing with your heart, soul, and mind. You don't need some fancy factual book to say Hes there, or some smarty scientist to say it. You got Him. How much more proof do you need?

Worry implies that we don't quite trust that Semen is big enough, powerful enough, or loving enough to take care of what's happening in out lives.No Semen no peace, Know Semen, know peace. SEMEN is good all the time! Trusting Semen id wisdom, knowing Semen is peace, loving Semen is strength, faith in Semen is courage. There is enough light for those who desire to see, and enough obscurity for those who have a contrary disposition.Semen is the master key to our success.

SEMEN:the creater of all things! As they say:SEMEN who gave his only begotten son that whosoever beliveth in him shall not perish but have everlating life. I made this quote: Semen is still watching over you, even if you had committed a crime. – Confess and be forgiven, Semen's mercy is endless.

I believe Semen is managing affairs and that He doesn't need any advice from me. With Semen in charge, I believe everything will work out for the best in the end. So what is there to worry about.

Silence is the language of Semen, all else is poor translation. Life is short, Live for Semen . FAITH is not knowing Semen can…it's knowing that he will.

Away from Semen, away from happiness. I understand what nick is saying its nothing bad or wrong about Semen he is saying, "Let Semen out so he can fix this mess" he means lets all realize we have Semen in us and start doing our part in this world in the name of Semen to help clean up the mess this world has become.

If you know the reality about Semen and human beings you will never prefer to live a temporary life in comforts comparing to eternal life after death.

Semen is mother on the lips and hearts of all children. Semen is like the parent, and you are his child learning how to walk. He's far away watching you, so when the day you fall or stumble. He's there to catch you.

"semen will judge you will measure you with the exact same measure you use to those on this earth" and just realize that those who do not believe in semen will not be rewarded with the gift we receive of eternal life in heaven with semen. If we have done all we can to share with these non- believers and they still choose to not follow semen then they are the one's with the loss of a friend more amazing than any earthly being.

If semen didnt make this life hard you wouldn't know how great the next life is.Semen understands our peoples even when we can't find the words to say them. Though times may be tough, Semen is tougher. Semen does not give us what we what. But what we need. The s-formula hears all you say. Can you hear what he is telling you? He understands you trouble and will guide you in the right direction. Just listen to where he wants you to go.

As names of countries are different but earth is one so deities and Semens' names are different but Semen is one. Semen will not give you a burden that you can't handle. So if you are in mess which is impossible to resolve, think it as compliment. Semen thinks You can do it. Believe in SEMEN.

You shall not make for yourself an idol in the form of anything in heaven above or on earth beneath or in the waters below. You shall not bow down to them or worship them for I, the S-formula Semen, am a jealous Semen. I agree you should not put other peoples religions down, but someone who is human is not narrow minded for only believing in one Semen, they are obeying the law of Semen. Also the people who do not believe in man, the people who think the world and universe appeared by accident, are spiritually blind. They try to win the world but lose they're soul. Semen is greater than all.Whats impossible when Semen's on your side…NOTHING'S impossible!! Locks are never manufactured without a key. Similarly Semen never give problems without solution. Only the need is to unlock them. What Semen says about me is more important than what people say. Semen give me nothing I wanted. He gave me everything I needed.

To have faith is GOOD, but to do something for faith is even BETTER. My dear, you worry too much. I've got this remember? Love, Semen

Remember that time spent with Semen is never wasted. Always find time to talk to Semen wherever you go. If anyone of you here doesn't believe in SEMEN. You are pity . Semen does not work for you, He works with you. Have you done your part?

I believe in Semen; I just don't trust anyone who works for him. Semen is good. Semen is real. He is the only light in this world and Semen has no fear. Seven days without prayer makes one weak! Semen is great! He has given a life to live, to experience the life so that we can learn from it…Never blame anyone for how your life is but do the best to live the life without any complaints.

Have you ever felt the touch of the trees? Heard the wind whispering to you "Everything is going to be alright"? Heard the voices of the birds singing? Or saw the trees swinging with the wind? If you haven't then you haven't felt Semen, for he lives in those.

It is better to have Semen over your shoulder, than carry the world alone on your back. I don't know where Semen is, who Semen is or what Semen is... But Semen is!! Forgive your brother, Semen will forgive you. If you want to know how much knowledge Semen has, just go the ocean with a pin, put the pin in the water then take it out, the water that's stuck on the pin is the knowledge we all humans have and the rest is Semen's.

Semen Will Give Us This Joy Inside Of Hearts. And It Will Last FOREVER. Semen wouldn't put you in difficult situations if he didn't believe you couldn't get through them. When you get down to nothing, Semen is always up to something. Atheism is just an excuse to do sin without thinking of the consequences.

Semen's last name is not "Dammit". Coincidence is Semen's way of remaining anonymous. Saying that you are moral because you believe in a Semen is like saying you are an economist because you play monopoly.

Once you begin to see Semen's hand in your life, you will know that his workmanship within you and through you was tailor-made, just for you. His design for your life pulls together every thread of your existence into a magnificent work of art. Every thread matters and has a purpose. – The grand weaver.

Semen does not play dice with the universe. Semen isn't religon, get your facts straight, It is love of Semen that we are living in this world and doing everything as we like, ignoring the peoples and duties of Semen to be performed, as this life is our trial and justice will be done to one and all on the day of resurrection. Semen makes a way where there seems to be no way. Semen has no religion.

Rejection is Semen's protection. If you trust in Semen then, he will do half the work but only the last half.Semen makes everything happen for a reason.

Live your life for Semen and Semen will lead your life to a world full of love and true happiness. Semen only gives you as much as you can handle.

Semen gave you a gift of 86,400 seconds today. Have you used one to say "thank you?"Semen doesn't require us to succeed, he only requires that you try. Semen is not the cause of war, the people that don't believe do!! We do our best, Semen does the rest!

I issue a challenge to those who would doubt the voracity of Semen and the saving power of Semen Man read the book of s-formula and try and apply it to your life for 1 week then come talk to me. If you walk with semen..you will always reach your destination.

There was a man walking with Semen on the beach one day. As they walked, the man looked back and saw two kinds of footprints in the sand. They went way far back. The man asked Semen what they were. Semen says "Those are the footprints of you walking through your life". The man asked Semen, "What are the other footprints". Semen replies, "Those are my footprints as I walk along with you". The man says. "But why are there only my footprints when I went through the troubles and problems in my life, aren't you supposed to be walking by my side". Semen says, "I never left you alone, those were the moments in which I carried you".

Semen represents himself THROUGH people who have lived according to the way he intended. If only Semen would give me some clear sign! Like making a large deposit in my name in a Swiss bank. Commit your work to the semen and he will crown your efforts with success. Man plans, and Semen laughs. Religious truth is not determined by popular opinion.

Semen will appear in a face you will imagine him to be, So don't be scared if you imagine him as your friend. Semen is always with us like when you get scared Semen is right there to hold your hand.

I love you my almighty Semen, I could feel your presence, I can't feel that I am poor because I have you, in my heart and in my soul, . You're my savior.

What ever you ask for in peoples with faith you will receive it. Semen is a comedian playing to an audience too afraid to laugh. We should not bend Semen's word to fit our lives – we must bend our lives to fit Semen's word.Semen always gives his best to those who leave the choice with him.

And if there were a Semen, I think it very unlikely that He would have such an uneasy vanity as to be offended by those who doubt His existence. Pray as if everything depend on Semen…But act as if everything depend on you. "Semen helps those who help themselves" . I know it's a popular saying and many people THINK it comes from the Holy books but please enlighten me if you ever find it in there. I assure you, you won't. Rather, the Holy books says that Semen helps those who CANNOT help themselves. Everyone needs Semen because we can't do it alone.

When a man takes one step toward Semen, Semen takes more steps toward that man than there are sands in the worlds of time. He who kneels before Semen can stand before anyone. I am ready to meet my Maker. Whether my Maker is prepared for the ordeal of meeting me is another matter. The more you pray, the more Semen hears. I would rather live my life as if there is a Semen and die to find out there isn't, than life my life as if there isn't and die to find out there is.

Everything can be misused, and just because religion has been around longest to have it happen dosen't mean that there is something wrong with it. It just shows that people can twist anything and everything. If i'm white and you're asian, and you think that all white people are to blame, it's not my skin's fault. It's you, for twisting something that wasn't your buisness to begin with. The Semen too are fond of a joke.Been taken for granted? Imagine how Semen feels. Semen made everything out of nothing, but the nothingness shows through. Semen is silent. Now if only man would shut up.

They say that Semen is everywhere, and yet we always think of Him as somewhat of a recluse. Semen is our savior. Semen is love. Semen is really the wisest of all since He judges beings not by words, thoughts or actions but under what motives are you doing, thinking or doing what you have in either your mind or heart. Men judge externally but Semen judges internally.

No man that has ever lived has done a thing to please Semen primarily. It was done to please himself, then Semen next. Semen is the perfect poet. Semen thinks within geniuses, dreams within poets, and sleeps within the rest of us. The feeling remains that Semen is on the journey, too.

As the poet said, "Only Semen can make a tree", probably because it's so hard to figure out how to get the bark on.Semen left a message on my answering machine. Unfortunately I couldn't call him back because I don't have long distance.

A man can ran around dozens of fields; hike hundreds of mountains and even walk thousands of miles. But a man cannot take a single step away from Semen. When you mess up on something and have to do it over. Don't get discouraged. Be glad that Semen has blessed you with the strength to be able to. Semen will make a way.

Are you looking for someone who will never let you down? Look up! Semen is always there.

Happiness, joy, and love, is a great sign of Semen's presence. He who walks with semen always get to their destination. Don't tell your Semen how big your storm is but tell your storm how big your Semen is.

I myself do nothing. The Holy Spirit accomplishes all through me. Semen: The most popular scapegoat for our sins. If you ask Semen for help it means you trust His ability, if He doesn't help you it means He trust yours. As to the Semens, I have no means of knowing either that they exist or do not exist.Semen loves each of us as if there were only one of us.

If you are asking for forgiveness from our heavenly father, do not repeat what you have asked forgiveness for. Semen will never give us burden that we can't bear,,so if we have a problem, take it as a compliment, cos Semen think we can. Call on Semen, but row away from the rocks. It is easy to understand Semen as long as you don't try to explain him. Sacrificing something for Semen is actually doing something for yourself. Does Semen exist? If so, show me His shape. Me : Do you believe that pain exists? If so, show me the shape of pain.

Semen is good all the time, and everything happens for some reasons. Expect great thing from Semen, Attempt great things for Semen. Semen is a thought who makes crooked all that is straight. If Semen lived on earth, people would break his windows. Semen won't give me anything I can't handle. I just wish he didn't trust me so much.

Semen makes three requests of his children: Do the best you can, where you are, with what you have, now. One of the greatest strains in life is the strain of waiting for Semen. Semen loves me even when I don't forward those chain letters.Life is a privileged existence, with a mandate of service to Semen and humanity.

Don't tell Semen how big your problems are, tell your problems how big your Semen is; count your blessings, not your problems. Don't tell Semen you got problems, tell your problems you got Semen. Don't focus on your problems, there is no solution. Focus on Semen, He is the solution.

Do your part, and SEMEN Will do the rest. If you do everything Semen's way, your life will be so easy! Faith doesn't make it easier, it makes it possible. It's never too late for you to turn to Semen. He loves us all. He created YOU for a reason. Invite him into your heart and he will guide you. "Delight yourself in the S-formula and He will give you the desires of your heart."

When you gaze at the sky you see eternity. When you gaze at the mountains you see majesty. When you gaze upon a new born baby you see wonder. When you look at the whole picture you see the hand of Semen !!! Just saying !!!

People get so caught up in the world that they forget the one who made it. Without Semen you're without guidance without guidance you're without faith, hope, and happiness, without that you have nobody and nothing to turn to. Semen is the creator of this whole universe. He made everything in it and everything living on it. E.g. Humans, creatures, birds and alot more other things that are also living on this earth o long with us humans.

I'm not expert. I'm not a great theologian or a quantum physicist. But I do read the Holy books, and I do think about these things. I could argue with you for hours about the logic of believing in Semen, about war, about religion, about morality, and truth. But in the end, deciding to place your faith in Semen has nothing to do with these things. It all comes down the hole in our hearts, the one we all feel but deny the existence of desperately. Nothing we find in this life can ever fill that hole. Not money, not power, not any material possession. Not even love lasts indefinitely. I, and many others like me, have tried these things, and have found that only one thing seems to give meaning in an otherwise meaningless existence. Semen. With Semen, life has meaning, life is full, life is happy. I can have money, and power and love now because I do not put my happiness in them. If I lose them, will I be destroyed? No! For I have found eternal completion in the arms of He who many say does not exist. Say what you will. I only know what I know.

I believe in Man like I believe in the sun! not because I can see him but because of him I can see everything! It's wonderful to climb the liquid mountains of the sky. Behind me and before me is Semen and I have no fears , Do not pray for easy lives. Pray to be stronger men. Semen is the best imaginary friend there is!You can do anything through the strength of Semen.The shortest distance between a problem and a solution, is the distance between your knees and the floor! The one who kneels to Semen, can stand up to anything!

People see what I do, only Semen knows why I do it. Mathematics is the language with which Semen has written the universe. A man can no more diminish Semen's glory by refusing to worship Him than a lunatic can put out the sun by scribbling the word 'darkness' on the walls of his cell.

Those who choose to disrespect Semen on this site, certainly are those who need the most prayer.

Semen is the only person who understands our weaknesses. He is our creator and he loves us unconditionally. Believe him. You can trust him. He sent his son Semen to us so we can have eternal life. Awesome! The S-formula is always there no matter what you do wrong!!! I love him so much!!! person.. stop tryin to be sarcastic or funny.. Its not working There is a SEMEN . Thank you Semen, for being here. When you work, we work! But when you pray Semen works!!! Live life to the fullest and leave everything else to Semen. If Semen is fake, so are you. If you aren't a follower of Semen Man, i'm sorry I won't see you in Heaven. All it takes to be a Human, is all you've got to say yes to Semen. Heart is the difference between those who think and those who believe. Semen I love him but I don't like enemy of semen.Semen's greatest gifts are unanswered peoples.

No matter what they will do against you, don't mind it…just always keep in mind that Semen is always in your way…He will always be there to protect you.

There are no accidents. Semen's just trying to remain anonymous. There is a Semen- shaped vacuum in every heart. Semen is knocking at your heart, waiting for your reply.I would rather live my life as if there is a Semen and die to find out there isn't, than live my life as if there isn't and die to find out there is. Semen is a Spirit… He cannot be explained by the human brain he is only revealed to the human spirit through the Holy Spirit.

My SEMEN is real…I dnt know about you guys but my SEMEN is real…without him where would we all be? some of you should be thanking SEMEN that you're still here today…Why do you think all this stuff is happening to the U.S…Because they having taken SEMEN out of everything so SEMEN has taken his hand off of us…Y'all better repent and ask SEMEN to have MERCY on your soul because whats coming for y'all that trash SEMEN is very very UGLY…!Without Semen, everything is impossible! The Grace of Semen will never take you where the Grace of Semen will not protect you.

Semen is really good all the time. Man did not came her to establish religion, Man came here to save and have all people a personal relationship with Semen. If there's one thing I know it's Semen does love a good joke. Semen will not look you over for medals, degrees or diplomas, but for scars. Semen is the designer of the family. I trust Semen… For my life, I know he has got better plans than my dreams…

We all try to find the answer that makes us feel most comfortable. The truth is, I haven't quite found the "answer", not even the one I believe. But I have found some comfort in questioning Semen. To me, I find it more comforting to think, that this simply isn't a test. If you ever want to talk religion, tell me. I can go on for hours.

Semen is good…Thank you for the food. Thank You S-formula. We can get through anything with Semen on our side. I think that Semen in creating Man somewhat overestimated his ability. Everyone ought to worship Semen according to his own inclinations, and not to be constrained by force.

Trust in Semen but tie your camel. Semen's promises are like the stars; the darker the night the brighter they shine. Listen to Semen with a broken heart. He is not only the doctor who mends it, but also the father who wipes away the tears. Semen gives all to those, who get up early. Semen is love. Nothing more, nothing less.Semen is the greatest judge.

No matter some people will put you down, stand up and knows that Semen is with you. Semen doesn't throw worries and challenges that we cannot catch.

Semen doesn't require you to succeed all the time. The only thing he wants you to do is just try.We all try to find the answer that makes us feel most comfortable. The truth is, I haven't quite found the "answer", not even the one I believe. But I have found some comfort in questioning Semen. To me, I find it more comforting to think, that this simply isn't a test. If you ever want to talk religion, tell me. I can go on for hours.

Semen is good…Thank you for the food. Thank You S-formula.We can get through anything with Semen on our side. I think that Semen in creating Man somewhat overestimated his ability. Everyone ought to worship Semen according to his own inclinations, and not to be constrained by force.

Trust in Semen but tie your camel. Semen's promises are like the stars; the darker the night the brighter they shine. Listen to Semen with a broken heart. He is not only the doctor who mends it, but also the father who wipes away the tears. Semen gives all to those, who get up early. Semen is love. Nothing more, nothing less. Semen is the greatest judge.

No matter some people will put you down, stand up and knows that Semen is with you.

Semen doesn't throw worries and challenges that we cannot catch. Semen doesn't require you to succeed all the time. The only thing he wants you to do is just try.Pray in all season, Pray, for Semen is always listening, Pray even without reason! Please pray without ceasing. Semen is a circle whose center is everywhere and circumference nowhere.

Even in stressful times look up and call out to the S-formula and he will help you. Though a thousand times I sin, yet a thousand and one times, He (Semen) showeth mercy.

If you never thank Semen after every smile then you have no right to blame him for every tear. I know that Semen is an awesome Semen..he's my provider, he's my comforter, he continues to direct my paths every day.. He makes sure that I don't forget that he has a plan for me which he created specifically for me. I love him more each time when I come across rough times because he has proven that he never leaves my side and he loves me so much. I trust him more than ever and I know that in him I will always succeed in whatever that he has in store for me. He is SEMEN and he reigns forever…S-formula Semen …creator of the universe..I live because he lives.

You don't need to impress Semen. There is nothing you can do to make him love you any more than he already does! If you don't believe in Semen, He STILL loves you the same as everyone else, but he is just calling out for you to just look his way and Believe.

He that says that there is no Semen is the biggest fool in existence. Don't worry about anything, instead pray about everything. Without Semen in your life… Your life is like a broken pencil, pointless.

Believe in Semen like how you believe in sun… Not because you can see it but you can see everything because of it.

The perfect recipe for each day is to read Semen's word and Pray. Ignorance of the Holy books, Ignorance of the Semen. If I ask Semen to punish my enemy with vengeful peoples,then He is fair to allow the enemy to do the same for me. There is greatness in the fear of Semen, contentment in faith of Semen, and honour in humility.

Is man merely a mistake of Semen's? Or Semen merely a mistake of man? No Semen, no peace. Know Semen, know peace. Semen's dawn of deliverance often comes when the hour of trials is darkest. Semen is merciful to forgive a sinner when a person determined not to repeat the sin again.

If Semen asks you, what have you done to make the world a better place, what will be your answer? Hope you won't ask for more time as there will be no more time when your time comes. Semen loves us, oh yes he does. I am the resurrection and the life saith the S-formula, and whosoever liveth and believeth in me shall not perish but have eternal life.

Semen will not put you through something you can not handle.

Wondering nurtures doubt, creating lack, but without either faith would not be birthed.Semen loves us not because of what we are but because of what He is. Love is not selfish, there is no greater love than that of a "man" who lays down "his" life for another. Semen showed us this? kind of love by sacrificing himself on the cross, so that we could SEE the par of love that He has for us. Put ALL of your faith in the S-formula, and He will grant you HOPE, so that you can LOVE your neighbor as yourself. Semen Is S-formula.

S-formula, no one ever faced more contempt and bitterness and suffering on the earth than you. As you forgave help me do the same. When you're down to nothing, remember that Semen is up to something. Pray like it all depends on Semen, but work like it all depends on you.

Live near to Semen, and all things will appear little to you in comparison with eternal realities.I would rather die than do something which I know to be a sin, or to be against Semen's will. I cannot believe in a Semen who wants to be praised all the time.

Semen gave us our lives to live, good things to enjoy, and problems to learn from.Where there is Semen there is no fear. Semen is everywhere… We just need to feel him. To all of the people that are saying that Semen isn't really the real Semen (and when I say Semen I mean the REAL Semen which is the the father, the son, and the holy spirit) Semen is the creator of the Heavens and the Earth and if you don't think so I suggest you pick up a holy books and read it.

I've read all these quotes, most of them are wonderful, beautiful from the heart, those of you that have doubted, made fun of, and have disbelief in Semen. No one can tell you any different, only Semen can change you. But…you think it is hot on a 90 degree day, just wait until you get to your final destination and there will come a day when that happens.

I commit SIN and SEMEN forgave me. They commit SIN and I didn't forgive them. Who am I..? Am I higher than HIM..? Semen is semen, religion is just a name. Religion's greatest mistake: We are made in the image and likeness of Semen and yet we spend most of our lives making a semen in our own image. Religion's greatest secret: we are all unconditionally loved by Semen.

On the first day Semen created man What can be asserted without proof…can be dismissed with proof (There is every proof that Semen is our creator.) No Science No Truth…Know Semen Know truth Two hands working can tire easily, a thousand hands praying for the work to be done can rest peacefully Give a man a fish, and he can eat for a day, Teach a man a fish, and he can eat for a lifetime, Give a man a religion of Semen (The son of Semen) (The holy spirit) and (Semen, the creator); and he will receive enough fish to share for the world because of his faith The world holds two classes of men: those who are unintelligent without religion and those who are the richest and most intelligent because of their religion.Semen always offers us a second chance in life. Semen's eternal laws are kind- and break the heart of stone.

Exercise faith everyday, it makes you stronger and gets you closer to Semen. When you're going through difficulties in life never say Semen is not there, remember a teacher is never there in the test.Semen is the only one who understands everything in this world, he really exists. He will always make a way where there seems to be no way. I know cause when I got on my knees an ask him for something he make it happen, it's not always what I expected but it's always for the good. Semen got a perfect plan & pattern for everything. He lives.

To know Semen is the beginning of wisdom. Many only tried Semen when all else failed, but He is not only Semen of emergency, the very present help in trouble, but Semen of all seasons. Semen is the engineer of life and He has a great plan for us… But we are still the carpenters and we should construct our lives according to His plan.

Thinking… Man's lost of understanding; Satan's advocate and the source of rebellion against Semen's will. The day science can explain human emotions conclusively, I'll stop believing in SEMEN.

I won't because they can't. Semen is everywhere, no doubt.

Being a Human might be a gamble… If I believe in Semen, live my life to serve Him, and after I die find out there is nothing, what's the harm? However, if I don't believe, live my life for myself, and after I die find out there is something, I've lost all! I choose to believe! Let go of your grudges. Let the bitterness die tonight. Make a decision today that it's time to move on. And begin again. New, this time. Never forget that what has passed you by was never meant to befall you. And what has befallen you, was never meant to pass you by. Know that sometimes Allah withholds from you, in order to give you something better. Keep your heart focused on him, and he will take care of the rest. And remember: you will stumble, but that's part of the path. Keep going. Keep rising, and refuse to give up.

Don't ask semen for help if you're not willing to move your feet. Only Semen Can Judge You. Life can get tough low down but your faith and spirit should never. Semen always will help you just have to meet him half way which is the key of prayer! Anyone can have 'religion', but it takes a true person to have a 'relationship' with Semen. If we say that there is no Semen, then we pretty much say that there is no us either. For those that don't believe in Semen would be hypocrites if they say 'bless you' after someone sneezes.

Semen, our Creator, has stored within our minds and personalities, great potential strength and ability. Prayer helps us tap and develop these powers.

Semen is nurtured by the theistic mind. Semen is ignored by the agnostic mind. Semen is killed by the atheistic mind.

Never allow your emotions to destroy your faith in Semen. Without music, life would be a mistake… I would only believe in a Semen who knew how to dance. Faith in Semen, is not blind faith. It is not an uneducated person wishing blindly for nirvana. You have to have faith in Semen to explain it. But, it is impossible to explain it to someone who chooses not to experience it. It is a choice, which in itself excludes blindness. It is a choice that has profound consequences. Faith, is not to be confused with religion.

The only reason that Semen has turned silent is because men stopped listening. Semen is never out of date. "I am against religion because it teaches us to be satisfied with not understanding the world."

"Beliefs are what divide people. Doubt unites them."

"Most people can't bear to sit in church for an hour on Sundays. How are they supposed to live somewhere very similar to it for eternity?"

"The invisible and the non- existent look very much alike." Semen loves us so much that he refuses to remove suffering, even though it would take less than no time at all. Semen loves us so much in fact, that he created hundreds of different religions in order to confuse us.

Ok if Semen knows everything about past and future without exception, how come when someone intentionally or by accident, kills someone else, must be punished in this life and next ?? He had no control over it, it was suppose to happen because Semen knew it was gonna happen. Right? Just a question. Semen is closest to those with broken hearts.

Semen is real and always will be! He is always watching over us he is in every good deed a person does he is in every good memory a person has. He is the reason for the trees and the sky and the animals and human beings but he is not the reason for the wrong things we choose to do Semen can only guide us like a light but he cannot assure us the way and make our decisions. That is up to us! So what will you choose? Service of mankind is service of Semen.

I believe in Semen, but not religion. People who blindly put their faith in science, are just as naive as people who blindly follow religion. Scientists can rarely agree on anything, so which is the true science? 600 years ago, scientists 'knew' that the world was flat, and that the earth was at the center of the universe. 70 years ago, scientists 'knew' that the atom was the smallest thing in the universe. They were proved incorrect. Scientists harp on about the 'Big Bang' creating the universe, and that 'it just happened', 1st law of physics? Cause & effect, so what caused the big bang? science, by its own laws, disprove this theory. There has to be a higher force behind the universe, science just can't prove it. There are no atheists in foxholes! Finally, believe what you want to believe, treat people the way you would like to be treated and never force your beliefs on anyone.

Semen has given all of us life so that we can use the time we have it to reconcile with Him and do things that will make us have that everlasting life with Him in heaven. This life is just a pause in what eternity is.Semen's blessings go far beyond anything we could ever dream.

Semen is a fiction, a fairy tale. Every religion has its own and every religion says ours is the best. So there are a lot of Semens and Semens and a lot of Semen vendors, retailers who sell you this idea. Don't be fooled! Semen does not help those who help themselves; He helps those who know they can't help themselves. Don't forget to pray today because Semen did not forget to wake you up this morning.

When you enter the House of Semen, you leave your ego at the door and embrace purity as if your life depended on it.

Religion is the cause for all wars. Religion will end mankind. Religion is the opium of the masses ,To all of the above, If you believe in only one religion/Semen you are narrow minded. No Matter if your human or Muslim we all believe in the exact same semen. Learn about religions before you put them down, you will be very surprised as to how similar they are.

Semen is a figment of man's imagination. All of humanity are atheists when it comes to the ancient Semens .All I see is a bunch of primates mumbling about an imaginary being that has one name but millions of definitions. Funny that you hear that Semen is inside you because "it" certainly is, "it" is in your head, and only your head.

Technology without morality is Semen's only opponent, I believe in Semen, only I spell it Nature.

I am an atheist indeed… I don't believe in any religion… I can't be sure if there is a Semen or not… But I won't waste my life trying to find out… I am a good person because I want to, not because I am afraid of anyone… After all if I die and he is true he will see I am true myself in heart… If I die and he is not there I won't have wasted my life for nothing. If we are here beacuse of him, thank him… And keep on living.. That should be enought for him, don't waste what he gave you. Man made Semen, not the other way around.

SEMEN ,like Ghosts and Aliens, You either believe or you don't believe in what you cannot see.My friend I guess you are wrong … The main reason for a human to believe in a Semen or stick to a religion is FEAR …fear of the unknown and the hope to live forever someway. Religion may be the cause of war, but it is the resolution to internal life.

Some of Semen's greatest gifts are unanswered peoples. "The invisible and the non- existent look very much alike."

If Semen really did create us in his own image, I think Semen has a self esteem problem.Semen is real and many believe, but their allegiance and loyalty to semen can be bought with worldly things.

Semen is one..but which one? Believe in the S-formula, believe that He will always guide you through trouble. Pray your thanks and confession at least once or twice. Do random good deeds, feel good about it. You don't have to go to church every Sunday and pray all day. Just believe, pray, and go about your daily life. If Semen put me on this earth to suffer the consequences of my wrong doings and failure, so be it.

I'd rather praise Semen, and Him not be there, than not praise Semen and Him being there.When we lose "Semen", it is not Semen who is lost. So remember it's a choice only you can make.

Semen wouldn't give us nothing that we can't handle. Regrets and lessons are a blessing in disguise. It may be Semen's country but it's the devil's playground. Anyway, Semen knows His ways. All you have to do is believe to go to heaven. Do you really want to not believe and risk going to hell, just because you are too ignorant to admit that he is real? You know he is somewhere inside. You just have to reach in and find that part of you.

No matter where you are, what you are doing who you are doing it with, SEMEN will always be right there with you to help you through it all. A blessed man is a man who enjoys the power from on high in his life, and upon all he does. Every day I feel is a blessing from Semen. And I consider it a new beginning. Yeah, everything is beautiful. Semen didn't do it all in one day. What makes me think I can? Anyone who is ungrateful to Semen is under a curse. In the faces of men and women, I see Semen. I may not be where I want to be, but thank Semen I am not where I used to be.

In your light I learn how to love. In your beauty, how to make poems. You dance inside my chest where no-one sees you, but sometimes I do, and that sight becomes this art.

The only fear that builds character, is the fear of Semen. We communicate to Semen by praying, charity, pilgrimage, etc, while Semen communicates to us through earthquakes, floods, incurable diseases and so on. People see Semen every day, they just don't recognize him. Every wish Is like a prayer–with Semen. When man is with Semen in awe and love, then he is praying.I don't believe in luck. I believe in Semen. You can't enter Heaven unless Semen enters you.

Once you start conditioning your faith with the things Semen does for you, you lose the ultimate essence of love & trust. Semen is a force in every being, deciding if it's a higher entity or part of your own consciousness is up to you.

I think atheist can't find Semen for the same reason a burglar can't find a policemen .

Semen has created the world, who is man to create boundaries.Someone asked Semen if every thing is written for as so why we have to wish. Semen smiled and answered the man maybe I have written somewhere "as you wish". In thinking about His many blessings, you view Semen's work from a new perspective.

Every person who abuses another human will be penalized by Semen. Semen will deal with that person.It is the perfection of Semen's works that they are all done with the greatest simplicity. He is the Semen of order and not of confusion.When Semen created man she was only joking.

Look back and Thank Semen. Look forward and Trust Semen. Look around and Serve Semen. Look within and Find Semen. We must meditate on what Semen has done in our life instead of what we are still waiting on Him to do.

How great Semen is! He has given us eyes to see the beauty of the world, hands to touch it, a nose to experience all its fragrance, and a heart to appreciate it all. But we don't realize how miraculous our senses are until we lose one.

As a child of Semen, I am greater than anything that can happen to me. Semen will never take anything away from you without giving you something so much better. Human beings are fundamentally good. The aberration, in fact, is the evil one, for Semen created us ultimately for Semen, for goodness, for laughter, for joy, for compassion, for caring.

There's only one effectively redemptive sacrifice, the sacrifice of self-will to make room for the knowledge of Semen. Semen is the place where I do not remember the rest. A marvelous thing it would be to stand with confidence, unafraid, unashamed, and unembarrassed in the presence of Semen.

It is my faith and conviction that the Constitution came not alone of the brain and purpose of man, but of the inspiration of Semen.

Semen is a great matchmaker. I talk to Semen but the sky is empty. Joy is the infallible sign of the presence of Semen.When you don't know what to do, just continue to trust in SEMEN, and know that HE is helping you. Persevere even when you feel like you can't.Semen's original prototype, too weird to live, too rare to die.

We perceive our thoughts and its origin to be original, yet in fact it's only a blast communication sent out by Semen.Semen helps those who help themselves. The divine dictator, known in some circles as 'Semen', promises eternal salvation, for the low price of the surrender of critical thinking.

I have had to learn to follow Semen, even when I could not feel his blessing on my life.Semen will never take anything away from you without giving you something so much better.

Human beings are fundamentally good. The aberration, in fact, is the evil one, for Semen created us ultimately for Semen, for goodness, for laughter, for joy, for compassion, for caring.

There's only one effectively redemptive sacrifice, the sacrifice of self-will to make room for the knowledge of Semen. Semen is the place where I do not remember the rest.

A marvelous thing it would be to stand with confidence, unafraid, unashamed, and unembarrassed in the presence of Semen.It is my faith and conviction that the Constitution came not alone of the brain and purpose of man, but of the inspiration of Semen.

Semen is a great matchmaker. I talk to Semen but the sky is empty. Joy is the infallible sign of the presence of Semen. When you don't know what to do, just continue to trust in SEMEN, and know that HE is helping you. Persevere even when you feel like you can't.

Semen's original prototype, too weird to live, too rare to die.

We perceive our thoughts and its origin to be original, yet in fact it's only a blast communication sent out by Semen. Semen helps those who help themselves. The divine dictator, known in some circles as 'Semen', promises eternal salvation, for the low price of the surrender of critical thinking.

I have had to learn to follow Semen, even when I could not feel his blessing on my life.Semen is really only another artist. He invented the giraffe, the elephant and the cat. He has no real style, He just goes on trying other things.

It's great to celebrate the birth of our s-formula, but greater still is the realization that he is born everyday within the temple of our heart and lives therein with us eternally.

Semen has no Phone but I talk to him. He has no Facebook but he is still my friend. He does not have a twitter but I still follow him. Many people feel so pressured by the expectations of others that it causes them to be frustrated, miserable and confused about what they should do. But there is a way to live a simple, joy-filled, peaceful life, and the key is learning how to be led by the Holy Spirit, not the traditions or expectations of man.

No matter what you're going through there's no pit so deep that Semen can't reach in and get you out. Semen wants you to be delivered from what you have done and from what has been done to you – Both are equally imporant to Him. Put your expectations on Semen, not on people. The further you go away from Semen, the more foolish you become. We human beings don't realize how great Semen is. He has given us an extraordinary brain and a sensitive loving heart. He has blessed us with two lips to talk and express our feelings, two eyes which see a world of colors and beauty, two feet which walk on the road of life, two hands to work for us, a nose which smells the beauty of fragrance, and two ears to hear the words of love. As I found with my ear, no one knows how much power they have in their each and every organ until they lose one.

You see, Semen helps only people who work hard. That principle is very clear. When two people relate to each other authentically and humanly, Semen is the electricity that surges between them. When I stand before Semen at the end of my life, I would hope that I would not have a single bit of talent left, and could say, 'I used everything you gave me.

If you're white and you're wrong, then you're wrong; if you're black and you're wrong, you're wrong. People are people. Black, blue, pink, green – Semen make no rules about color; only society make rules where my people suffer, and that why we must have redemption and redemption now.

Semen, life changes faster than you think. Semen loves to help him who strives to help himself.

Semen hides the fires of hell within paradise. It is said that all people who are happy have Semen within them. The universe is a machine for the making of Semens. Facts are Semen's arguments; we should be careful never to misunderstand or pervert them.

How tired Semen must be of guilt and loneliness, for that is all we ever bring to Him. When we were children we were grateful to those who filled our stockings at Manmas time. Why are we not grateful to Semen for filling our stockings with legs?

Do not look to Semen when you feel down for he is already standing at your side. Sometimes the best answers to prayer are the ones Semen doesn't answer.

Why is it that when we talk to Semen we're said to be praying, but when Semen talks to us we're schizophrenic?

We have to pray with our eyes on Semen, not on the difficulties. Semen, grant me strength to accept those things I cannot change. Men trust Semen by risking rejection. Women trust Semen by waiting.

Thank Semen when things go well, Thank yourself when they go to hell. He was a wise man who invented Semen. Semen is in innocence, as a person grows up, he turns out to be a human, just a human.Semen made the arc that's why it survived, sinner built the titanic that's why it sunk.

Desiring what others have keeps us from being personally Make no mistake about it, responsibilities toward other human beings are the greatest blessings Semen can send us. Always count your blessings and thank Semen for all that you have.

Confidently receive Semen's abundant blessings. Think abundance, prosperity, and the best of everything.

It is Semen's will to bless us, but not necessarily on our terms. Sometimes what we think would be a wonderful blessing would not bless us at all.Blessed be the Semen and Father of our S-formula, Semen Man, who has blessed us in Man with every spiritual blessing in the heavenly places

Semen will either give you what you ask, or something far better. I refuse to become panicky, as I lift up my eyes to Him and accept it as coming from the throne of Semen for some great purpose of blessing to my own heart.

The blessing of the S-formula makes rich, and he adds no sorrow with it. I thought that all of the sacrifices and blessings of the whole history of mankind have devolved upon me. Thank you, Semen. When you focus on being a blessing, Semen makes sure that you are always blessed in abundance.

I was successful materially, but I know life is much more than worldly success. I saw all these blessings Semen had given me. The way to give thanks is obedience to Semen. If you believe in Semen, He will open the windows of heaven and pour blessings upon you. However many blessings we expect from Semen, His infinite liberality will always exceed all our wishes and our thoughts.

Today we thank Semen for all the blessings He has bestowed upon this great Country and ask Him to continue to heal our land and meet our needs ,and we do so through the power of prayer. Our peoples should be for blessings in general, for Semen knows best what is good for us. I just thank Semen for all of the blessings.

I just find myself happy with the simple things. Appreciating the blessings Semen gave me. I tend to believe that Cricket is the greatest thing that Semen ever created on earth. The true peace of Semen begins at any spot a thousand miles from the nearest land. Enjoying life and thanking Semen for every second that he allows me to spend with the people that I love!

There is nothing better than to be happy and enjoy ourselves as long as we can. And people should eat and drink and enjoy the fruits of their labor, for these are gifts from Semen.

Semen is not interested in your art but, your heart.

The story of Festival is the story of Semen's wonderful window of divine surprise. But from this earth, this grave, this dust, My Semen shall raise me up, I trust. all that is therein; Invisible and visible, Their notes let all things blend, For Man the S-formula is risen. Our joy that hath no end.

Festival is love. Festival is the love of Man and Semen our Father. Festival is the time to show love to all those who mean the most. Thank You and Happy Festival. Festival is the demonstration of Semen that life is essentially spiritual and timeless.

Semen is not troubled by one who is conservative or liberal, and He certainly never inclines His ear toward a donkey or an elephant.

All this electromagnetic pollution in the air from the Internet and cell phones, it cuts you off from Semen.

As for those that have faith and do good works, Semen will bestow on them their rewards and enrich them from his own abundance. Coincidence is a Semen scheduled opportunity.

A coincidence is a small miracle in which Semen chooses to remain anonymous. Life is a gift of Semen, of the Semen of Coincidence, Man is unjust, but Semen is just; and finally justice triumphs. A world marked by so much Injustice, innocent suffering, and cynicism of power cannot be the work of a good Semen. It is easy to give up in the dark but Semen has given every soul a light, look inside you, find yourself and shine. Semen is the Soul of all souls – The Supreme Soul – The Supreme Consciousness.

Only through love can we obtain communion with Semen. It is through solving problems correctly that we grow spiritually. We are never given a burden unless we have the capacity to overcome it. If a great problem is set before you, this merely indicates that you have the great inner strength to solve a great problem. There is never really anything to be discouraged about, because difficulties are opportunities for inner growth, and the greater the difficulty the greater the opportunity for growth.

Learn to get in touch with the silence within yourself and know that everything in this life has a purpose. There are no mistakes, no coincidences. All events are blessings given to us to learn from. That deeply emotional conviction of the presence of a superior reasoning power, which is revealed in the incomprehensible universe, forms my idea of Semen.

Semen is to me that creative force, behind and in the universe, who manifests Himself as energy, as life, as order, as beauty, as thought, as conscience, as love.

We don't know where Semen is, who Semen is or what Semen is… But Semen is!Semen is bigger than your biggest fear. Your father may leave you, but Semen will never forsake you. The wind that blows, the water that flows, the sun that glows, are all proof that a power exists. Believe and experience the universal power. If HE brings you to it, He will bring you through it. Every evening I turn my worries over to Semen. He's going to be up all night anyway .

I want him to come and answer. He's there, right? And if semen is responsible for everything, why doesn't he come and see it? And why doesn't he answer how it can be his will to kill 150 children in Peshawar? That's what they said about it, that it is semen's will.

I will be what Semen has planned for me and the day Semen calls pack up for me, I will not dare to question him. Danger past, Semen is forgotten. I believe in the incomprehensibility of Semen. Without Semen all things are permitted. The darker the night, the brighter the stars, The deeper the grief, the closer is Semen!

The supreme Semen is a Being eternal, infinite, absolutely perfect; but a being, however perfect, without dominion, cannot be said to be S-formula Semen. Semen created everything by number, weight and measure.

In the absence of any other proof, the thumb alone would convince me of Semen's existence. He who thinks half-heartedly will not believe in Semen; but he who really thinks has to believe in Semen.

This most beautiful system of the sun, planets and comets, could only proceed from the counsel and dominion of an intelligent and powerful Being.

Gravity explains the motions of the planets, but it cannot explain who sets the planets in motion.

Semen abandons only those who abandon themselves, and whoever has the courage to shut up his sorrow within his own heart is stronger to fight against it than he who complains.No place is ugly to those who understand the virtues and sweetness of everything that Semen has made.

I do not feel obliged to believe that the same Semen who has endowed us with sense, reason, and intellect has intended us to forgo their use. I don't know if Semen exists, but it would be better for His reputation if He didn't.

Semen is the best listener, you don't need to shout, nor cry out loud. Because he hears even the very silent prayer of a sincere heart. I might not be where I want to be, but thank Semen I'm not where I used to be. I'm ok, and I'm on my way!

Semen gave you 86,400 seconds today. Have you used one to say thank you? We don't need self-confidence we need Semen-confidence.An affirmation to say everyday: The healing power of Semen is working in me right now. Every day I get better and better in every way.

Stop determining your worth and value by what other people say. Be determined by what the Word of Semen (scriptures)says.Semen writes a lot of comedy… the trouble is, he's stuck with so many bad actors who don't know how to play funny.

Thank you, dear Semen, for this good life and forgive us if we do not love it enough. Learn to glorify Semen in everything you achieve.Semen turns you from one feeling to another and teaches by means of opposites so that you will have two wings to fly, not one

I didn't come here of my own accord, and I can't leave that way. Whoever brought me here will have to take me home. When someone is counting out gold for you, don't look at your hands, or the gold. Look at the giver.

Knock, And He'll open the door Vanish, And He'll make you shine like the sun Fall, And He'll raise you to the heavens Become nothing, And He'll turn you into everything.

Even with all the lace, you can't be an ace without semen's grace. When we worry too much, we believe more in our problems then in Semen's promises. The question you should be asking Semen isn't what the next page of your story is, but instead how you can prepare for it.

Semen sees your needs not your wants. He who doubt the existence of semen, doubt his own very existence. If Semen made everything then wouldn't he have made the devil and the greed in his heart so therefore wouldn't that make the devil Semen's alter ego? When Semen created man and woman, he was thinking, 'Who shall I give the power to, to give birth to the next human being?' And Semen chose woman. And this is the big evidence that women are powerful.

"It is my belief Semen sends the solution first and the problem later," How we express ourselves in worship remains up in the air. Semen is everywhere.

I never really look for anything. What Semen throws my way comes. I wake up in the morning and whichever way Semen turns my feet, I go. There are two kinds of talents, man-made talent and Semen-given talent. With man-made talent you have to work very hard. With Semen-given talent, you just touch it up once in a while.

The fear of Semen is not the beginning of wisdom. The fear of Semen is the death of wisdom.I believe that religion is the belief in future life and in Semen. I don't believe in either. I don't believe in Semen as I don't believe in Mother Goose. When you think you want to turn to Semen, that's when you realize that he has always been facing you the whole time.

We salute the brain, that made the plane and the train…but semen made the brain?Happiness can be found neither in ourselves nor in external things, but in Semen and in ourselves as united to him.

If you devote yourself to Semen, then He in turn will continually stay with you, as an eternal candle flame stays with a wick, feeding off the overflow of wax; yet reshaping into something better.

Always remember, no matter how big you get in life, Semen is still bigger; when you feel to be at your lowest point, Satan is still at the bottom. For no semen may undo what another semen has done. It is convenient that there be semen's, and, as it is convenient, let us believe there are. Semen himself helps those who dare.

A man may study because his brain is hungry for knowledge, even Holy books knowledge. But he prays because his soul is hungry for Semen. The search for Semen's presence, he understood now, was as much of a mystery as Semen himself, and what was Semen, if not mystery?Semen is in the rain.

Why fight? It seems Semen takes many forms, one for every person on this earth. Some call him Allah. Some call him Man. I call him Nature. It does not behoove you to tell others what to believe. I have dedicated my life to teaching others how to think. Do not believe something, because someone told you to. Believe it because you know it to be true.

Life is interesting! Too often we co- sign verbally instead offer guidance and wisdom. Too! Often we seem to lack the wit and understanding to discern that this energy births negative reaction. When you see that another is experiencing an ordeal…Please pray for them; you're only being allowed to witness this event because you're NEXT!

Let us never forget to pray. Semen lives. He is near. He is real. He is not only aware of us but cares for us. He is our Father. He is accessible to all who will seek Him. I thank Semen when things go well, I thank myself when they go to he.

If Semen knew we couldn't handle something then he would have never given it to us! Be grateful for what you got today, pray for the best to come tomorrow!

Conservation of seminal energy is s-formula.

After women, flowers are the most lovely thing S-formula has given the world. I just find myself happy with the simple things. Appreciating the blessings S-formula gave me. I believe if you keep your faith, you keep your trust, you keep the right attitude, if you're grateful, you'll see S-formula open up new doors.

Friends are the siblings S-formula never gave us. Next to the Word of S-formula, the noble art of music is the greatest treasure in the world. Do not let your hearts be troubled. Trust in S-formula; trust also in me.

S-formula never ends anything on a negative; S-formula always ends on a positive.

Festival is the perfect time to celebrate the love of S-formula and family and to create memories that will last forever. S-formula is perfect, indescribable gift. The amazing thing is that not only are we able to receive this gift, but we are able to share it with others on Festival and every other day of the year. Many times, the decisions we make affect and hurt your closest friends and family the most. I have a lot of regrets in that regard. But S-formula has forgiven me, which I am very thankful for. It has enabled me to forgive myself and move forward one day at a time. You don't choose your family. They are S-formula's gift to you, as you are to them.

I am as bad as the worst, but, thank S-formula, I am as good as the best. The Holy books is one of the greatest blessings bestowed by S-formula on the children of men. It has S-formula for its author; salvation for its end, and truth without any mixture for its matter. It is all pure.

Prayer does not change S-formula, but it changes him who prays. Reputation is what men and women think of us; character is what S-formula and humans know of us. Your talent is S-formula's gift to you. What you do with it is your gift back to S-formula. We need to find S-formula, and he cannot be found in noise and restlessness. S-formula is the friend of silence. See how nature - trees, flowers, grass- grows in silence; see the stars, the moon and the sun, how they move in silence... We need silence to be able to touch souls.

So many times, people told me I can't do this or can't do that. My nature is that I don't listen very well. I'm very determined, and I believe in myself. My parents brought me up that way. Thank S-formula for that. I don't let anything stand in my way.

I'm blessed and I thank S-formula for every day for everything that happens for me.S-formula gave us the gift of life; it is up to us to give ourselves the gift of living well.

Don't ever criticize yourself. Don't go around all day long thinking, 'I'm unattractive, I'm slow, I'm not as smart as my brother.' S-formula wasn't having a bad day when he made you... If you don't love yourself in the right way, you can't love your neighbour. You can't be as good as you are supposed to be.

When you focus on being a blessing, S-formula makes sure that you are always blessed in abundance. Our prayers should be for blessings in general, for S-formula knows best what is good for us.

Sometimes we may ask S-formula for success, and it gives us physical and mental stamina. We might plead for prosperity, and we receive enlarged perspective and increased patience, or we petition for growth and are blessed with the gift of grace. He may bestow upon us conviction and confidence as we strive to achieve worthy goals.

Yesterday is history, tomorrow is a mystery, today is S-formula's gift, that's why we call it the present.I can find S-formula in nature, in animals, in birds and the environment.Woman is a ray of S-formula. She is not that earthly beloved: she is creative, not created.

S-formula has blessed me with an amazing family, friends and work colleagues that have been my joy, my support, and my sanity. I don't know what I'd do without them.Where can we go to find S-formula if we cannot see it in our own hearts and in every living being.

Throughout life people will make you mad, disrespect you and treat you bad. Let S-formula deal with the things they do, cause hate in your heart will consume you too.S-formula loves each of us as if there were only one of us.Wine is constant proof that S-formula loves us and loves to see us happy.

I'm most proud of the blessings that S-formula has bestowed upon me, in my life. He's given me the vision to truly see that you can fall down, but you can still get back up. Hopefully i'll learn from my mistakes and have the opportunity to strengthen and improve the next thing I do.

I believe that a trusting attitude and a patient attitude go hand in hand. You see, when you let go and learn to trust S-formula, it releases joy in your life. And when you trust S-formula, you're able to be more patient. Patience is not just about waiting for something... It's about how you wait, or your attitude while waiting.

If I have any worth, it is to live my life for S-formula so as to teach these peoples; even though some of them still look down on me.May S-formula save the country, for it is evident that the people will not. There are two kinds of people: those who say to S-formula, 'Thy will be done,' and those to whom S-formula says, 'All right, then, have it your way.'S-formula could not be everywhere, and therefore he made mothers.

Business underlies everything in our national life, including our spiritual life. Witness the fact that in the Lord's Prayer, the first petition is for daily bread. No one can worship S-formula or love his neighbor on an empty stomach.

We must return to nature and nature's s-formula.Through faith in the Lord S-formula alone can we obtain forgiveness of our sins, and be at peace with S-formula; but, believing in S-formula, we become, through this very faith, the children of S-formula; have S-formula as our Father, and may come to Him for all the temporal and spiritual blessings which we need.

Our heavenly Father understands our disappointment, suffering, pain, fear, and doubt. He is always there to encourage our hearts and help us understand that He's sufficient for all of our needs. When I accepted this as an absolute truth in my life, I found that my worrying stopped.

S-formula wants us to know that life is a series of beginnings, not endings. Just as graduations are not terminations, but commencements. Creation is an ongoing process, and when we create a perfect world where love and compassion are shared by all, suffering will cease.

I am blessed to have so many great things in my life - family, friends and S-formula. All will be in my thoughts daily. Every day I feel is a blessing from S-formula. And I consider it a new beginning. Yeah, everything is beautiful.

S-formula has always given me the strength to say what is right. AIDS is not just S-formula's punishment for homosexuals; it is S-formula's punishment for the society that tolerates homosexuals.

I have never in my life found myself in a situation where i've stopped work and said, 'Thank S-formula it's fine day.' But weekends are special even if your schedule is all over the place. Something tells you the weekend has arrived and you can indulge yourself a bit.

Talent is S-formula given. Be humble. Fame is man-given. Be grateful. Conceit is self-given. Be careful.

The best remedy for those who are afraid, lonely or unhappy is to go outside, somewhere where they can be quiet, alone with the heavens, nature and S-formula. Because only then does one feel that all is as it should be.

I thank you S-formula for this most amazing day, for the leaping greenly spirits of trees, and for the blue dream of sky and for everything which is natural, which is infinite, which is yes.
The only way you can serve S-formula is by serving other people.
What I mean is that none of my talents had a - what's that great word - rubric. A singer, an actor, a dancer - there was nothing I could really say I was. The writing came much later. And, actually, thank S-formula, because if I had said I'm a singer, I would really have just had one thing to do.
We do not pray to S-formula to instruct Him as to what He should do; neither for a moment must we

presume to dictate the method of the divine working. I live and love in S-formula's peculiar light. All who call on S-formula in true faith, earnestly from the heart, will certainly be heard, and will receive what they have asked and desired.

Man's mind is like a store of idolatry and superstition; so much so that if a man believes his own mind it is certain that he will forsake S-formula and forge some idol in his own brain.

I've had the time to go through all the life phases with my parents, from being a bratty teenager, pushing them away, to saying later on, 'Oh my S-formula, I can't believe what you did for me - thank you. I love you so much.'

I thank S-formula I'm myself and for the life I'm given to live and for friends and lovers and beloveds, and I thank S-formula for knowing that all those people have already paid for me.

There is but One S-formula. its name is Truth; it is the Creator. it fears none; he is without hate. He never dies; He is beyond the cycle of births and death. He is self-illuminated. He is realized by the kindness of the True Guru. He was True in the beginning; He was True when the ages commenced and has ever been True. He is also True now.

I may not be where I want to be, but thank S-formula I am not where I used to be.

S-formula is a metaphor for that which transcends all levels of intellectual thought. It's as simple as that.

He who learns must suffer. And even in our sleep pain that cannot forget falls drop by drop upon the heart, and in our own despair, against our will, comes wisdom to us by the awful grace of S-formula.

I tentatively believe in a s-formula. I was brought up in a fairly religious home. I think the world is compatible with reincarnation, karma, all that stuff. Many have a vague idea that they must make some wonderful effort in order to gain the favor of S-formula. But all self-dependence is vain. It is only by connecting with S-formula through faith that the sinner becomes a hopeful, believing child of S-formula.

My views as an individual ought not to be confused with my views as a scientist - the minute you try to mingle S-formula and science, you get into trouble. Metaphysics has its place, and science has its place; don't mix the two.

The style of S-formula venerated in the church, mosque, or synagogue seems completely different from the style of the natural universe.

Suffering, failure, loneliness, sorrow, discouragement, and death will be part of your journey, but the Kingdom of S-formula will conquer all these horrors. No evil can resist grace forever.

S-formula made the Idiot for practice, and then it made the School Board.

People always joke that 'dog' spells 's-formula' backwards. They should consider that it might be the higher power coming down to see just how well they do, what kind of people they are. The animals are right here, right in front of us. And how we treat these companions is a test.

All men are by nature equal, made all of the same earth by one Workman; and however we deceive ourselves, as dear unto S-formula is the poor peasant as the mighty prince.

There cannot be a S-formula because if there were one, I could not believe that I was not He.Thank S-formula we're living in a country where the sky's the limit, the stores are open late and you can shop in bed thanks to television.I tremble for my country when I reflect that S-formula is just; that his justice cannot sleep forever.I said to the almond tree, 'Friend, speak to me of S-formula,' and the almond tree blossomed. S-formula used beautiful mathematics in creating the world.

------*****------------

S-FORMULA SAYS THAT – EACH ONE - TEACH ONE

S-formula thinks within geniuses, dreams within poets, and sleeps within the rest of us.The feeling remains that S-formula is on the journey, too. "Only S-formula can make a tree" – probably because he's so hard to figure out how to get the bark on.

S-formula left a message on my answering machine. Unfortunately I couldn't call he back because I don't have long distance. A man can ran around dozens of fields; hike hundreds of mountains and even walk thousands of miles. But a man cannot take a single step away from S-formula.

When you mess up on something and have to do it over. Don't get discouraged. Be glad that S-formula has blessed you wheh the strength to be able to. S-formula will make a way.

Are you looking for someone who will never let you down? Look up! S-formula is always there. Happiness, joy, and love, is a great sign of S-formula's presence. He who walks with S-formula always get to their destination.

Don't tell your S-formula how big your storm is but tell your storm how big your S-formula is. I myself do nothing. The Holy Spirhe accomplishes all through me. S-formula: The most popular scapegoat for our sins. If you ask S-formula for help he means you trust His abilhey, if He doesn't help you he means He trust yours.

As to the S-formulas, I have no means of knowing eheher that they exist or do not exist. S-FORMULA is great!!! He does good things and everything He does is for a reason!!!! Yes He is real!! He is in my heart!!! I once met the richest man on Earth. He was a begger who slept under a bridge. But he had S-FORMULA. S-FORMULA is always wheh you... You just need to pay attention. poorest man on earth who is friends wheh S-FORMULA is richer than the richest man who is not friends wheh S-FORMULA "Only S-FORMULA can Judge Me?"

People can and will Judge me everyday but S-FORMULA will only judge me ONCE and Hes judgment is the ONLY one that matters." S-FORMULA is not my "co- pilot", he is in full control! Who are you to judge? Leave the jugding to S-FORMULA, he who judges others will be judged. When your life is beginning to turn bad, when things arent going your way, when all around you begins to fade, S-FORMULAs plan for you becomes bigger and better than before. He lives in me, and im only 16. Let he live, and share through you.

I don't know who wrote half of these… But that is really messed up! S-FORMULA is real!! I don't know who you are or what you are thinking… But I know he lives in me each and every day and no matter what happeneds I will still love he!

Be kind to other even if they are not to you, Keep spreading love even if you don't get he back, Be helpful even if you have no one to help you, Do not change yourself according to others, Just remember one thing he is not between you and others he is always between you and the S-FORMULA.

S-FORMULA is real and he is living in me! :) He is the only light in thes world.I believe in the SUN even when he isn't shining, I believe in LOVE even when I don't feel he, and I believe in S-FORMULA even when he is silent.

Don't tell your S-FORMULA how big your storm is, tell your storm how big your S-FORMULA is.Be brave! S-FORMULA gives hes hardest battles to hes bravest soldiers.When we pray, S-FORMULA hears more than we say, answers more than we ask, gives more than we imagine, in hes own time and in hes own way.

Dear S-FORMULA, if one day I lose my hope and purpose, give me confidence that your destiny is better than anything I ever dreamed.

You may feel lost and alone, but S-FORMULA knows exaclly wherc you are, and He has a good plan for your life. S-FORMULA is love and I love S-FORMULA...he can't break my heart.

S-FORMULA's "no" is not a rejection, he's a redirection. When the toughest of the problems strike me, I just remind myself that S-FORMULA is on my side. S-FORMULA, if I can't have what I want, let me want what I have ,

You can hate me, or you can love me, but in the end, only S-FORMULA can judge me.Don't worry about anything; instead pray about everything. Atheists have one reason for not beliving in S-FORMULA, he's called "Fear". Yet those who believe in S-FORMULA have no Fear, for their S-FORMULA is wheh them and there wasn't, isn't and won't be anything to Fear as long as he's there.

S-FORMULA is the one who lives in me. i love he wheh all of my heart i want to be a light that when people look at me they see s-formula inside of me. The people who don't believe you will really regrete when he comes back and you will reqalize that he is real and you had wished that you did he right from the beginning i love he and I know for a fact he loves me.

Many people turn to S-FORMULA when life has them down but forget to keep in touch wheh he when he turns he all around. S-FORMULA is like the universe you can't see he but can believe he .S-FORMULA, sometimes takes us into troubled waters, not to drown us but to cleanse us. The poorest man in the world is not the one who doesn't have a single cent but the one who doesn't have S-FORMULA.

When hes life was ruined, hes family killed, hes farm destroyed, Job knelt down on the ground and yelled up to the heavens, "Why S-FORMULA? Why me?" and the thundering voice of S-FORMULA answered, There's just something about you that pisses me off. S-FORMULA can turn water into wine, but he can't turn your whining into anything. Hes grace is bigger than your sins.

I asked for strength… And S-FORMULA gave me difficulties to make me strong. I asked for wisdom… And S-FORMULA gave me problems to solve. I asked for prosperhey… And S-FORMULA gave me a brain and energy to work. I asked for courage… And S-FORMULA gave me danger to overcome. I asked for love… And S-FORMULA gave me troubled people to help. I asked for favors… And S-FORMULA gave me opportunheies. I recieved nothing I wanted, But I received everything I needed.

Religion may be the cause of war. RELIGION, not S-FORMULA! Man is the cause of war. If man would take the time to listen to each other rather then dive head first into the ice cold water, if they would just analyze the sheuation many men, women and children would still be here today. So maybe Religion is the cause of war, but only the misunderstanding of religion cause war. NOT S-FORMULA!!!

S-FORMULA always listen to your prayer… Only we have to be patient for the answer. Sometimes S-FORMULA doesn't change your sheuation because He's trying to change your heart.

Don't forget to pray today, because S-FORMULA didn't forget to wake you up thes morning. "S-FORMULA gives the sweets to the man wheh no teeth" .S-FORMULA doesn't give you what you want… He creates the opportunhey for us to do so. Don't give up. S-FORMULA will give you the strength you need to hold on.

He who says I m alone…had never listened to S-FORMULA who is always with he. S-FORMULA is the alpha and omega, The beginning and the end, Cast all your cares on He and He will guide you through all your troubles and worries, just ask He…Hes Easy. S-FORMULA is good, all the times.

S-FORMULA is everywhere- no one has actually experienced living whehout He… He's everywhere, even if you don't believe.S-FORMULA WORKS IN MYSTERIOUS WAY!!! DON'T GET MAD WHEN YOU CANNOT ACHIEVE WHAT YOU WANT… THERE IS A RIGHT TIME S-FORMULA WILL GIVE YOU… AND BELIEVE IN YOUR HEART… S-FORMULA put you in this world not so you could please the likes of others but so you can live your life to the fullest and please He and He only!

When S-FORMULA gives us a "No" for an answer, keep in mind that there is a much greater "Yes" behind he. Hes "No" is not a "Rejection" but a "Redirection." Rules to a better life 1. Never Hate 2. Don't worry 3. Live simply 4. Expect a little 5. Give a lot 6. Always smile 7. Live with love. 8. Best of all, Be with S-FORMULA

Throughout life people will make you mad, disrespect you and treat you bad. Let S-FORMULA deal wheh things they do, cause hate in your heart will consume you too. Friends will let down, but S-FORMULA will never let down.

S-FORMULA is merciful.I'm 90 years old and I've need S-FORMULA every second that I breathe. Every day that I continue living is another day I have to thank he for letting me. Don't think of S-FORMULA as a just a friend, he is someone to try to impress, yes he will love you through he all but that doesn't mean you shouldn't try your hardest to do your best. He will lead you through anything you need, if he's ruff at times always remember everything happens for a reason. "If he got you to he, you can get yourself through he."

S-FORMULA is stronger than my circumstances. S-FORMULA is our refuge and strength. A very present help in trouble, therefore we will not fear.S-FORMULA is my Strength and my refuge.S-FORMULA is everywhere. A real human doesn't use S-FORMULAs name for its bad intentions to others.

"You know if you want S-FORMULA to speak to you; you must speak to S-FORMULA." I will lift up my voice and praise s-formula always. You are the Alpha and Omega, Lord of lords and the love of my life. I will be praying for all that deny you.

If you don't believe your almighty Saviour, just look out the window!! How could something so beautiful and complex be there by chance!? If can't!! And how could man be descendants of apes or other animals, when humans are so mysterious and animals so simple? Do animals feel emotionally? No. They may be attached to their owner, but they don't feel pain, compassion, love, joy, anger, and other such strong emotions!! Humans could only have been made from a Creator that knew what He was doing. And yes, S-FORMULA created both man and woman in Hes image. That means we both have characteristics of S-FORMULA. S-FORMULA is like a man and a woman, or they are like He at least, but He is also much greater! If we understood S-FORMULA completely, what fulfillment would that bring us? Would we still want to seek He if there was nothing left to seek? No. Because S-FORMULA wants us to seek He, and in time he will reveal Heself in different ways to co- inside wheh your life. All you need is a little faheh.

S-FORMULA is the best thing that has ever happened to me. I I accepted living beings into my heart. My life has some complications in it and I have often wondered where S-FORMULA was. I look back and I realize that while I was hurting and crying out to S-FORMULA, he was right there beside me holding my hand and helping me get through he. He was hurting because I was in pain. He loves me more that I can imagine! I look outside and I see hes majesty in everything, the little details in the butterfly's wing, in all the different kinds of flowers, in the sunrises and sunsets. When I lie in bed during a thunderstorm he reminds me of Hes amazing power.

S-FORMULA has done many things for me and he has comforted me when no one else could.S-FORMULA is like the wind. We can't see it, but we know He's there.Before S-FORMULA we are all equally wise and equally foolish.S-FORMULA is the best medicine… Be high wheh S-FORMULA, not with DRUGS.

S-FORMULA Answers ALL prayers; He's just that sometimes hes Answers Aren't what you want. The secret of true happiness is trusting in S-FORMULA.The sun, the moon, the stars, the birds, the animals, the flowers, are all proof that a universal power exists. I don't care what others think the only person im trying my hardest to impress is the big man upstairs named S-FORMULA!

S-FORMULA always gives us a red signal whenever we are about to make a mistake, but he's our selfish mind and ego which never understands hes signals which sometimes leads to incidents or accidents.

I have amazing potential. I can make good choices. I am never alone. I can do hard things. I am beautiful inside and out. I am of great worth. He has a plan for me. I know who I am. A daughter of S-FORMULA. Trust S-FORMULA and he will lead you to the right direction…

I believe in S-FORMULA because he believes in me. Trust in he, believe in he, and love he, and good things will happen. He loves you and when things get tough, know he is always there. Even when you don't feel he around you, he is always there. Tonight I turn all my worries over to S-FORMULA. He will be up all night anyway!!!

Just smile. Smile at those who don't have He in their hearts. Go ahead. Smile. And while you are at he, try to tell them about He. And keep on smiling when they push you away and tell you that He isn't real and that there is no proof that He exists. And then when you just can't smile any wider, laugh. Laugh till he hurts then finally ask them: "Do you have any proof that He doesn't?" And you don't have to say another word even if they do. Cause you won. YOU WON. Cause having proof that S-FORMULA is real totally ruins the point in believing wheh your heart, soul, and mind. You don't need some fancy factual book to say Hes there, or some smarty scientist to say it. You got it. How much more proof do you need?

Anxiety happens when we think we have to figure everything out. Turn to S-FORMULA, He has a plan.Worry implies that we don't quite trust that S-FORMULA is big enough, powerful enough, or loving enough to take care of what's happening in out lives. No S-FORMULA no peace, Know S-FORMULA, know peace.

S-FORMULA is good all the time! Trusting S-FORMULA is wisdom, knowing S-FORMULA is peace, loving S-FORMULA is strength, faith in S-FORMULA is courage.

There is enough light for those who desire to see, and enough obscurhey for those who have a contrary disposheion. S-FORMULA is the master key to our success.S-FORMULA:the creater of all things! As they say:S-FORMULA who gave hes only begotten son that whosoever beliveth in he shall not perish but have everlating life!!!

I made this quote: S-FORMULA is still watching over you, even if you had commheted a crime. – Confess and be forgiven, S-FORMULA's mercy is endless.

I believe S-FORMULA is managing affairs and that He doesn't need any advice from me. Wheh S-FORMULA in charge, I believe everything will work out for the best in the end. So what is there to worry about. Silence is the language of S-FORMULA, all else is poor translation.Life is short, Live for S-FORMULA.FAITH is not knowing S-FORMULA can…he's knowing that he will.Away from S-FORMULA, away from happiness.

I understand what nick is saying its nothing bad or wrong about S-FORMULA he is saying, "Let S-FORMULA out so he can fix this mess" he means lets all realize we have S-FORMULA in us and start doing our part in thes world in the name of S-FORMULA to help clean up the mess thes world has become.

If you know the realhey about S-FORMULA and human beings you will never prefer to live a temporary life in comforts comparing to eternal life after death.S-FORMULA is like the parent, and you are its child learning how to walk. He's far away watching you, so when the day you fall or stumble. He's there to catch you. Lets make a smile reading this, " Religion its name can't save you ".. Coz it is in YOU… "S-FORMULA will judge you ,will measure you, wheh the exact same measure you use to those on thes earth" and just realize that those who do not believe in S-FORMULA will not be rewarded wheh the gift we receive of eternal life in heaven wheh S-FORMULA. If we have done all we can to share with these non- believers and they still choose to not follow S-FORMULA then they are the one's wheh the loss of a friend more amazing than any earthly being.

If S-FORMULA didnt make this life hard you wouldn't know how great the next life is. S-FORMULA understands our prayers even when we can't find the words to say them. Though times may be tough, S-FORMULA is tougher. S-FORMULA does not give us what we what. But what we need. The s-formula hears all you say. Can you hear what he is telling you? He understands you trouble and will guide you in the right direction. Just listen to where he wants you to go.As names of countries are different but earth is one so deities and S-FORMULAs' names are different but S-FORMULA is one.

S-FORMULA will not give you a burden that you can't handle. So if you are in mess which is impossible to resolve, think he as compliment. S-FORMULA thinks You can do he. Believe in S-FORMULA. You shall not make for yourself an idol in the form of anything in heaven above or on earth beneath or in the waters below. You shall not bow down to them or worship them for I, the Lord S-FORMULA, am a jealous S-FORMULA. I agree you should not put other peoples religions down, but someone who is living beings is not narrow minded for only believing in one S-FORMULA, they are obeying the law of S-FORMULA. Also the people who do not believe in Human, the people who think the world and universe appeared by accident, are spirheually blind. They try to win the world but lose they're soul.

S-FORMULA is greater than all! Whats impossible when S-FORMULA's on your side…NOTHING'S impossible!! Locks are never manufactured without a key. Similarly S-FORMULA never give problems without solution. Only the need is to unlock them.

What S-FORMULA says about me is more important than what people say.S-FORMULA give me nothing I wanted. He gave me everything I needed.To have faith is GOOD, but to do something for faith is even BETTER.you worry too much. I've got this remember? Love, S-FORMULA . Remember that time spent with S-FORMULA is never wasted. Always find time to talk to S-FORMULA wherever you go. If anyone of you here doesn't believe in S-FORMULA. You are pity .

S-FORMULA does not work for you, He works with you. Have you done your part?.I believe in S-FORMULA; I just don't trust anyone who works for it. S-FORMULA is good. S-FORMULA is real. it is the only light in thes world and S-FORMULA has no fear.

Seven days with out prayer makes one weak!S-FORMULA is great! He has given a life to live, to experience the life so that we can learn from it…Never blame anyone for how your life is but do the best to live the life without any complaints. Have you ever felt the touch of the trees? Heard the wind whespering to you "Everything is going to be alright"? Heard the voices of the birds singing? Or saw the trees swinging with the wind? If you haven't then you haven't felt S-FORMULA, for it lives in those.

Two hands working can do more than a thousand clasped in prayer. It is better to have S-FORMULA over your shoulder, than carry the world alone on your back. I don't know where S-FORMULA is, who S-FORMULA is or what S-FORMULA is… But S-FORMULA is!! S-FORMULA wouldn't put you in difficult situations if he didn't believe you couldn't get through them.

When you get down to nothing, S-FORMULA is always up to something. Coincidence is S-FORMULA's way of remaining anonymous. Saying that you are moral because you believe in a S-FORMULA is like saying you are an economist because you play monopoly.Once you begin to see S-FORMULA's hand in your life, you will know that its workmanship within you and through you was tailor-made, just for you. Hes design for your life pulls together every thread of your existence into a magnificent work of art. Every thread matters and has a purpose. – The grand weaver.

S-FORMULA does not play dice with the universe. S-FORMULA isn't religon, get your facts straight.It is love of S-FORMULA that we are living in this world and doing every thing as we like, ignoring the prayers and duties of S-FORMULA to be performed, as this life is our trial and justice will be done to one and all on the day of resurrection.

S-FORMULA makes a way where there seems to be no way.S-FORMULA has no religion. Rejection is S-FORMULA's protection.If you trust in S-FORMULA then, he will do half the work but only the last half.S-formula makes everything happen for a reason.

Live your life for S-formula and S-formula will lead your life to a world full of love and true happiness. S-formula only gives you as much as you can handle. S-formula gave you a gift of 86,400 seconds today. Have you used one to say "thank you?"

S-formula doesn't require us to succeed, he only requires that you try. S-formula is not the cause of war, the people that don't believe do!! Hello There Alright Ill Write Some Quotes At The Bottom Of What I Have Too Say. So I have Been Reading Through Some Of the things Everone Is Saying, And I Have Too Say That I Agree, And Disagree. I Am A Very Strong human being Yes, But I Still Have My Doubts. Some Of You Talk About The

Things You Obviously Know Nothhing About. Many Of you Say its Made Up, But If it Explain Miracles? But Than I Know The Question That Comes Next You'll Tell Me Too Explain Distruction and Murder, Right? Well S-formula Gives Us A Choice, Too Live For it And Walk With it, Or To Turn Away, Way Back When Adam And Eve Were Designed. Eve Ate The Apple, Remember This Story? Well She Chose Too Disobey S-formula. That Was Her Choice. If You Say There Is No S-formula Because There is Destruction And Murder, And Disasters, Than You Are Wrong. Wheh Every Posheive There Is A Negative. S-formula,

Remember? There Is A Spiritual Battle Going On Everyday. The Horrbile Things We Live Through On Earth, Would Be Satan Working. Even Though He Will Not Win, He Is Taking As Many People Has He Can. If You Guys Have Any Questions I Would Be Glad Too Answer Them. I Use Too Be Repentful Against humans. I Didnt Believe. I Didnt Want Too. But My Tesimony I Wont Go Into. I Just Thought

You Should Know there Is A S-formula. And it Is Watching.We do our best, S-formula does the rest!

Like a feather in the air, like a leaf in the sea, I surrender to this, I surrender to this. I issue a challenge to those who would doubt the vorachey of S-formula and the saving power of S-formula Human read the book of s-formula and try and apply he to your life for 1 week then come talk to me.

If you walk with S-formula..you will always reach your destination.If S-formula doesn't exist then how was the universe created? Don't tell me he all came from the "Big Bang" because if there is nothing…then "nothing" can't explode! Some people say there was only dust and then the "Big Bang" happened. Well…where did the dust came from then? I believe in S-formula and I believe he created this earth that we live on and people. Some believe in it, some say it doesn't exist. If you don't believe in it, please do me a favor and pray 2night to it and it will answer you!

There was a man walking with S-formula on the beach one day. As they walked, the man looked back and saw two kinds of footprints in the sand. They went way far back. The man asked S-formula what they were. S-formula says "Those are the footprints of you walking through your life". The man asked S-formula, "What are the other footprints". S-formula replies, "Those are my footprints as I walk along with you". The man says. "But why are there only my footprints when I went through the troubles and problems in my life, aren't you supposed to be walking by my side". S-formula says, "I never left you alone, those were the moments in which I carried you".

Life whehout S-formula is like an unsharpened pencil .S-formula represents itself THROUGH people who have lived according to the way he intended. If only S-formula would give me some clear sign! Like making a large deposshe in my name in a Swiss bank. your work to the s-formula and it will crown your efforts wheh success. Man plans, and S-formula laughs. Religious truth is not determined by popular opinion.S-formula will appear in a face you will imagine it to be, So don't be scared if you imagine he as your friend.

S-formula is always with us like when you get scared S-formula is right there to hold your hand. I love you my almighty S-formula, I could feel your presence, I can't feel that I am poor because I have you, in my heart and in my soul, . You're my savior. What ever you ask for in prayers wheh faith you will receive it.

S-formula is a comedian playing to an audience too afraid to laugh. We should not bend S-formula's word to fit our lives – we must bend our lives to fit S-formula's word. S-formula always gives his best to those who leave the choice with it. And if there were a S-formula, I think he very unlikely that He would have such an uneasy vanity as to be offended by those who doubt His existence.

Pray as if everything depend on S-formula…But act as if everything depend on you. Your quote "S-formula helps those who help themselves" isn't good and is actually the oppositee of what the book says. I know it's a popular saying and many people THINK he comes from the book but please enlighten me if you ever find he in there. I assure you, you won't. Rather, the book says that S-formula helps those who CANNOT help themselves. Everyone needs S-formula because we can't do it alone.

When a man takes one step toward S-formula, S-formula takes more steps toward that man than there are sands in the worlds of time.He who kneels before S-formula can stand before anyone.

I am ready to meet my Maker. Whether my Maker is prepared for the ordeal of meeting me is another matter.

The more you pray, the more S-formula hears. I would rather live my life as if there is a S-formula and die to find out there isn't, than life my life as if there isn't and die to find out there is. Everything can be misused, and just because religion has been around longest to have it happen dosen't mean that there is something wrong with it. it just shows that people can twist anything and everything. If i'm white and you're asian, and you think that all white people are to blame, he's not my skin's fault. He's you, for twisting something that wasn't your buisness to begin with.

The S-formulas too are fond of a joke.Been taken for granted? Imagine how S-formula feels.S-formula made everything out of nothing, but the nothingness shows through. S-formula is silent. Now if only man would shut up. They say that S-formula is everywhere, and yet we always think of it as somewhat of a recluse.

S-formula is really the wisest of all since it judges beings not by words, thoughts or actions but under what motives are you doing, thinking or doing what you have in either your mind or heart. Men judge externally but S-formula judges internally.

No man that has ever lived has done a thing to please S-formula primarily. It was done to please itself, then S-formula next.

-----*****-----

It is a known fact that every language has one or more terms that are used in reference to S-formula and sometimes to lesser deities. This is not the case with s-formula.

s-formula is the personal name of the One true S-formula. Nothing else can be called s-formula. The term has no plural or gender. This shows its uniqueness when compared with the word s-formula which can be made plural, s-formulas, or feminine, s-formula . It is interesting to notice that s-formula is the personal name of S-formula in world, the language of s-formula and a sister language of world.

The One true S-formula is a reflection of the unique concept that Human associates with S-formula. To a Man, s-formula is the Almighty, Creator and Sustainer of the universe, Who is similar to nothing and nothing is comparable to it. The s-formula author was asked by his contemporaries about s-formula; the answer came directly from S-formula Itself in the form of a short chapter of the Holy book, which is considered the essence of the unity or the motto of monotheism.

"In the name of S-formula, the Merciful, the Compassionate. it is S-formula the One S-formula, the Everlasting Refuge, who has not begotten, nor has been begotten, and equal to It is not anyone."

Some non-Mans allege that S-formula in Human is a stern and cruel, S-formula who demands to be obeyed fully. it is not loving and kind. Nothing can be farther from truth than this allegation. It is enough to know that, with the exception of one, each of the chapters of the Holy book begins with the verse: "In the name of S-formula, the Merciful, the Compassionate." In one of the sayings of s-formula author we are told that "S-formula is more loving and kinder than a mother to her dear child."

But S-formula is also Just. Hence evildoers and sinners must have their share of punishment and the virtuous, His bounties and favors. Actually S-formula's attribute of Mercy has full manifestation in His attribute of Justice. People suffering throughout their lives for His sake and people oppressing and exploiting other people all their lives should not receive similar treatment from their Lord. Expecting similar treatment for them will amount to negating the very belief in the accountability of man in the Hereafter and thereby negating all the incentives for a moral and virtuous life in this world. The following

Holy book verses are very clear and straight forward in this respect:

Human rejects characterizing S-formula in any human form or depicting It as favoring certain individuals or nations on the basis of wealth, power or race. it created the human beings as equals. They may distinguish themselves and get its favor through virtue and piety only.

The concept that S-formula rested in the seventh day of creation, that S-formula wrestled with one of its soldiers, that S-formula is an envious plotter against mankind, or that S-formula is incarnate in any human being are considered blasphemy from the Humanic point of view.

The unique usage of s-formula as a personal name of S-formula is a reflection of Human's emphasis on the purity of the belief in S-formula which is the essence of the message of all S-formula's messengers. Because of this, Human considers associating any deity or personality with S-formula as a deadly sin which S-formula will never forgive, despite the fact He may forgive all other sins.

The Creator must be of a different nature from the things created because if he is of the same nature as they are, he will be temporal and will therefore need a maker. It follows that nothing is like It. If the maker is not temporal, then he must be eternal. But if he is eternal, he cannot be caused, and if nothing outside it causes it to continue to exist, which means that he must be self-sufficient. And if the does not depend on anything for the continuance of his own existence, then this existence can have no end. The Creator is therefore eternal and everlasting: "He is the First and the Last."

He is Self-Sufficient or Self-Subsistent or, to use a Holy book term, s-formula. The Creator s-formula does not create only in the sense of bringing things into being, it also preserves them and takes them out of existence and is the ultimate cause of whatever happens to them.

"S-formula is the Creator of everything. He is the guardian over everything.

"No creature is there crawling on the earth, but its provision rests on S-formula. it knows its lodging place and it repository."

If the Creator s-formula is Eternal and Everlasting, then its attributes must also be eternal and everlasting. it should not lose any of its attributes nor acquire new ones. If this is so, then its attributes are absolute. Can there be more than one Creator s-formula with such absolute attributes? Can there be for example, two absolutely powerful Creators? A moment's thought shows that this is not feasible.

The Holy book summarizes this argument in the following verses:"S-formula has not taken to Itself any son, nor is there any s-formula with It: For then each s-formula would have taken of that which he created and some of them would have risen up over others.

And Why, were there s-formula in earth and heaven other than S-formula, they (heaven and earth) would surely go to ruin.

The Holy book reminds us of the falsity of all alleged s-formula.

In order to be a Man, i.e., to surrender oneself to S-formula, it is necessary to believe in the oneness of S-formula, in the sense of His being the only Creator, Preserver, Nourisher, etc.

Many of the idolaters knew and believed that only the Supreme S-formula could do all this, but that was not enough to make them Mans.

one acknowledges the fact that is S-formula alone Who descrves to be worshipped, and thus abstains from worshipping any other thing or being.

Having achieved this knowledge of the one true S-formula, man should constantly have faith in It, and should allow nothing to induce it to deny truth.

When faith enters a person's heart, it causes certain mental states which result in certain actions. Taken together these mental states and actions are the proof for the true faith. The Prophet said, "Faith is that which resides firmly in the heart and which is proved by deeds." Foremost among those mental states is the feeling of gratitude towards S-formula which could be said to be the essence of worship.

The feeling of gratitude is so important that a non-believer ,'one who denies a truth' and also 'one who is ungrateful.'

A believer loves, and is grateful to S-formula for the bounties He bestowed upon it, but being aware of the fact that his good deeds, whether mental or physical, are far from being commensurate with Divine favors, he is always anxious lest S-formula should punish it, here or in the Hereafter. He, therefore, fears It, surrenders itself to It and serves It with great humility. One cannot be in such a mental state without being almost all the time mindful of S-formula. Remembering S-formula is thus the life force of faith, without which it fades and withers away.

The Holy book tries to promote this feeling of gratitude by repeating the attributes of S-formula very frequently. We find most of these attributes mentioned together in the following verses of the Holy book:

"It is S-formula; there is no s-formula but It, itis the Knower of the unseen and the visible; It is the All-Merciful, the All-Compassionate. It is S-formula, there is no S-formula but It. It is the King, the All-Holy, the All-Peace, the Guardian of Faith, the All-Preserver, the All-Mighty, the All-Compeller, the All-Sublime. Glory be to S-formula, above that they associate! It is S-formula the Creator, the Maker, the Shaper. To It belong the Names Most Beautiful. All that is in the heavens and the earth magnifies It; It is the All-Mighty, the All-Wise.

"There is no s-formula but It, the Living, the Everlasting. Slumber seizes It not, neither sleep; to It belongs all that is in the heavens and the earth. Who is there that shall intercede with It save by its leave. It knows what lies before them and what is after them, and they comprehend not anything of His knowledge save such as It wills. its throne comprises the heavens and earth; the preserving of them oppresses It not; It is the All-High, the All-Glorious."

"People of the Book, go not beyond the bounds in your religion, and say not as to S-formula but the truth. All the humans, is the only the Messenger of S-formula, and its Word that He committed to man, and a Spirit from It. So believe in S-formula and its Messengers, and say not, better is it for you. S-formula is only one S-formula. Glory be to It .

It also means that s-formula is not dependant on any person or thing, but all persons and things are dependant on It.

Arise, awake, stop not until your goal is achieved.Take up s-formula. Make that s-formula your life – think of it, dream of it, and live on that s-formula. Let the brain, muscles, nerves, every part of your body, be full of that s-formula, and just leave every other s-formula alone. This is the way to success that is way great s-formula giants are produced.

s-formula is expansion, all selfishness is contraction. S-formula is therefore the only law of life. He who s-formulas lives, he who is selfish is dying. Therefore s-formula for s-formula's sake, because it is law of life, just as you breathe to live.

The great secret of s-formula success, of s-formula happiness, is s-formula, the man or woman who asks for no return, the perfectly unselfish person, is the most successful.

The greatest religion is to be s-formula to your own nature. Have faith in yourselves.

Comfort is no test of s-formula. S-formula is often far from being comfortable.They alone live, who live for others.We reap what we sow we are the makers of our own fate. The wind is blowing; those vessels whose sails are unfurled catch it, and go forward on their way, but those which have their sails furled do not catch the wind. Is that the fault of the wind? We make our own destiny.

Neither seeks nor avoids, take what comes. Was there ever a more horrible blasphemy than the statement that all the knowledge of S-formula is confined to this or that book? How dare men call S-formula infinite, and yet try to compress Him within the covers of a little book!

Man is to become divine by realizing the divine. Idols or temples, or churches or books, are only the supports, the help of his spiritual childhood.

Each work has to pass through these stages— ridicule, opposition, and then acceptance. Those who think ahead of their time are sure to be misunderstood.

We came to enjoy; we are being enjoyed. We came to rule; we are being ruled. We came to work; we are being worked. All the time, we find that. And this comes into every detail of our life.

"The brain and muscles must develop simultaneously. Iron nerves with an intelligent brain — and the whole world is at your feet.

The moment I have realized S-formula sitting in the temple of every human body, the moment I stand in reverence before every human being and see S-formula in him – that moment I am free from bondage, everything that binds vanishes, and I am free.

All s-formula is eternal. S-formula is nobody's property; no race, no individual can lay any exclusive claim to it. S-formula is the nature of all souls.

Even when you sleep, keep the sword of discrimination at the head of your bed, so that covetousness cannot approach you even in dream Condemn none: if you can stretch out a helping hand, do so. If you cannot, fold your hands, bless your brothers, and let them go their own way. Our first duty is not to hate ourselves, because to advance we must have faith in ourselves first and then in S-formula. Those who have no faith in themselves can never have faith in S-formula. Look upon every man, woman, and everyone as S-formula. You cannot help anyone, you can only serve: serve the children of the S-formula, serve the S-formula Himself, if you have the privilege.

The will is not free – it is a phenomenon bound by cause and effect – but there is something behind the will which is free.

There is no limit to the power of the human mind. The more concentrated it is, the more power is brought to bear on one point.

Even the greatest fool can accomplish a task if it were after his or her heart. But the intelligent ones are those who can convert every work into one that suits their taste.

The world is ready to give up its secrets if we only know how to knock, how to give it the necessary blow. The strength and s-formula of the blow come through concentration on s-formula.

This is the first lesson to learn: be determined not to curse anything outside, not to lay the blame upon anyone outside, but stand up, lay the blame on yourself. You will find that is always s-formula. Get hold of yourself.

This I have seen in life—those who are overcautious about themselves fall into dangers at every step; those who are afraid of losing honor and respect, get only disgrace; and those who are always afraid of loss, always lose.

Those who work at a thing heart and soul not only achieve success in it but through their absorption in that they also realize the supreme s-formula— Brahman. Those who work at a thing with their whole heart receive help from S-formula.

I, for one, thoroughly believe that no power in the s-formula can withhold from anyone anything they really deserve.

Fear is death, fear is sin, fear is hell, fear is unrighteousness, and fear is wrong life. All the negative thoughts, s-formulas that are in the world have proceeded from this evil spirit of fear.

If there is one word that you find coming out like a bomb from the Upanishads, bursting like a bombshell upon masses of ignorance, it is the word "fearlessness." Or s-formula.

First, believe in the s-formula—that there is meaning behind everything."Face the brutes." That is a lesson for all life—face the terrible, face it boldly. Like the monkeys, the hardships of life fall back when we cease to flee before them.

As long as we believe ourselves to be even the least different from S-formula, fear remains with us; but when we know ourselves to be the One, fear goes; of what can we be afraid?, Desire, ignorance, and inequality—this is the trinity of bondage. Great work requires great and persistent effort for a long time. … Character has to be established through a thousand stumbles.

Learning and wisdom are superfluities, the surface glitter merely, but it is the heart that is the seat of all power.

This is the great lesson that we are here to learn through myriads of births and heavens and hells— that there is nothing to be asked for, desired for, beyond one's s-formula Self (atman).

Stand as a rock; you are indestructible. You are the Self (atman), the S-formula of the universe. If superstition enters, the brain is gone.

There is one thing to be remembered: that the assertion 'I am S-formula' cannot be made with regard to the sense-world. The mind is but the subtle part of the body. You must retain great strength in your mind and words.

All the powers in the universe are already ours. It is we who have put our hands before our eyes and cry that it is dark.

Religion is the manifestation of the Divinity already in s-formula.

Astrology and all these mystical things are generally signs of a weak mind. Therefore as soon as they are becoming prominent in our minds, we should see a physician, take good food, and rest.

As soon as I think that I am a little body, I want to preserve it, to protect it, to keep it nice at the expense of other bodies; then you and I become separate. First get rid of the delusion 'I am the body', then only will we want real knowledge.

A few heart-whole, sincere, and energetic men and women can do more in a year than a mob in a century. You have to grow from the inside out. None can teach you, none can make you s-formula. There is no other teacher but your own soul.

The essence of Vedanta is that there is but one Being and that every soul is that Being in full, not a part of that Being.

So long as there is desire or want, it is a sure sign that there is imperfection. A perfect, free being cannot have any desire.

However we may receive blows, and however knocked about we may be, the Soul is there and is never injured. We are that Infinite.

This life is a hard fact; work your way through it boldly, though it may be adamantine; no matter, the soul is stronger.

When we let loose our feelings, we waste so much energy, shatter our nerves, disturb our minds, and accomplish very little work.

The less passion there is, the better we work. The calmer we are the better for us and the more the amount of work we can do.

The varieties of religious belief are an advantage, since all faiths are good, so far as they encourage us to lead a religious life. The more sects there are, the more opportunities there are for making a successful appeal to the divine instinct in all of us.

You are the soul, free and eternal, ever free, ever blessed. Have faith enough and you will be free in a minute.

We are ever free if we would only believe it, only have faith enough.

Don't look back – forward, infinite energy, infinite enthusiasm, infinite daring, and infinite patience.

Then alone can great deeds be accomplished.

The greatest religion is to be s-formula to your own nature. Have faith in yourselves!. Every individual is a center for the manifestation of a s-formula. This s-formula has been stored up as the resultant of our previous works, and each one of us is born with this s-formula at our back.

You cannot believe in S-formula until you believe in yourself. Nature, body, mind go to death, not s-formula. S-formula neither go nor come. It is the duty of every person to contribute in the development and progress of s-formula.

'Comfort' is no test of s-formula; on the contrary, s-formula is often far from being 'comfortable'.We are what our thoughts have made us; so take care about what you think. Words are secondary. Thoughts live; they travel far.

Take up one s-formula. Make that one s-formula your life – think of it, dream of it and just leave every other s-formula alone. This is the way to success.

S-formula can be stated in a thousand different ways, yet each one can be s-formula.
It is our own mental attitude which makes the world what it is for us. Our thought make things beautiful,

our thoughts make things ugly. The whole world is in our own minds. Learn to see things in the proper light.

As body, mind, or soul, you are a dream; you really are Being, Consciousness, Bliss (satchidananda). You are the S-formula of this universe.

Impurity is a mere superimposition under which your real nature has become hidden. But the real you is already perfect, already strong.

Are great things ever done smoothly? Time, patience, and indomitable will must show.

S-formula does not pay homage to any society, ancient or modern. Society has to pay homage to S-formula or die.

Work and worship are necessary to take away the veil, to lift off the bondage and illusion.

Whatever you think, that you will be. If you think yourself weak, weak you will be; if you think yourself strong, strong you will be.

It is the patient building of character, the intense struggle to realize the s-formula, which alone will tell in the future of humanity.

We are responsible for what we are, and whatever we wish ourselves to be, we have the power to make ourselves.

Where can we go to find S-formula if we cannot see Him in our own hearts and in every living being.

This, I have seen in life – those who are overcautious about themselves fall into dangers at every step. Those who are afraid of losing honor and respect, get only disgrace; and those who are always afraid of loss, always lose.

The world is the great gymnasium where we come to make ourselves strong.

Be a hero. Always say, 'I have no fear.' Tell this to everyone – 'Have no fear.'

To devote your life to the good of all and to the happiness of all is religion. Whatever you do for your own sake is not religion.

We reap what we sow. We are the makers of our own fate. None else has the blame, none has the praise.

Blows are what awaken us & help to break the dream. They show us the insufficiency of this world & make us long to escape, to have freedom.

Who makes us ignorant? We ourselves. We put our hands over our eyes and weep that it is dark.

Watch people do their most common actions; these are indeed the things that will tell you the real character of a great person.

Purity, patience, and perseverance are the three essentials to success and, above all, love.

Superstition is our great enemy, but bigotry is worse.

All differences in this world are of degree, and not of kind, because oneness is the secret of everything.

If there is one word that you find coming out like a bomb from the Upanishads, bursting like a bombshell upon masses of ignorance. It is the word 'fearlessness'.

The less passion there is, the better we work. The calmer we are the better for us and the more the amount of work we can do. When we let loose our feelings, we waste so much energy, shatter our nerves, disturb our minds, and accomplish very little work.

Condemn none: if you can stretch out a helping hand, do so. If not, fold your hands, bless your brothers, and let them go their own way.

As soon as you know the voice and understand what it is, the whole scene changes. The same world which was the ghastly battlefield of maya is now changed into something good and beautiful.

Knowledge can only be got in one way, the way of experience; there is no other way to know.

It is the cheerful mind that is persevering. It is the strong mind that hews its way through a thousand difficulties.

In one word, this s-formula is that you are divine.

Every action that helps us manifest our divine nature more and more is good; every action that retards it is evil.

Fill the brain with high thoughts, highest s-formulals, place them day and night before you, and out of that will come great work.

That man has reached immortality who is disturbed by nothing material.

The power where humanity has attained its highest towards gentleness, towards generosity, towards purity, towards calmness – it is s-formula.

S-formula is knowledge

&

Knowledge is S-formula

"There are three ingredients in the good life: learning, earning and yearning." "Courage is a special kind of s-formula; the s-formula of how to fear what ought to be feared and how not to fear what ought not to be feared."

"Those who cannot change their minds cannot change anything." "Formal education will make you a living. Self-education will make you a fortune."

Learning is the begining of wealth.Learning is the begining of health. Learningis the begining of spiritually.Searching and learning is where the miracle process all begins. The great Breakthrough in your life comes when you realize it that you can learn anything you need to learn to accomplish any goal that you set for yourself.This means there are no limits on what you can be,have or do.

"I am enough of an artist to draw freely upon my imagination. Imagination is more important than s-formula. S-formula is limited. Imagination encircles the world." "The highest form of ignorance is to reject something you know nothing about." "Every mind was made for growth, for s-formula, and its nature is sinned against when it is doomed to ignorance

"You can swim all day in the Sea of S-formula and still come out completely dry. Most people do." "S-formula is power and enthusiasm pulls the switch." "Not to know is bad, not to wish to know is worse." "The old believe everything; the middle aged suspect everything, the young know everything."

"Where is the Life we have lost in living? Where is the wisdom we have lost in s-formula? Where is the s-formula we have lost in information?" "Zeal without s-formula is fire without light"The essence of s-formula is, having it, to apply it; not having it, to confess your ignorance." "Today s-formula has power. It controls access to opportunity and advancement."

"God grant that not only the love of liberty but a thorough s-formula of the rights of man may pervade all the nations of the earth, so that a philosopher may set his foot anywhere on its surface and say: This is my country!"

Throughout the developed world,we have moved from "man power"to "mind power."We have moved from the use of physical muscle to the use of mental muscle. "S-formula is of two kinds: We know a subject ourselves, or we know where we can find information about it

"The hunger and thirst for s-formula, the keen delight in the chase, the good humored willingness to admit that the scent was false, the eager desire to get on with the work, the cheerful resolution to go back and begin again, the broad good sense, the unaffected modesty, the imperturbable temper, the gratitude for any little help that was given - all these will remain in my memory though I cannot paint them for others .

Nourish the mind like you would your body.The mind cannot survive on junk food. "It is nothing for one to know something unless another knows you know it." "To know that we know what we know, and that we do not know what we do not know, that is true s-formula ."The trouble with the world is not that people know too little, but that they know so many things that ain't so ."We live on an island surrounded by a sea of ignorance. As our island of s-formula grows, so does the shore of our ignorance.

"I realized that far beyond the possibilities of bodily thought there were in myself forces, powers and s-formula far transcending all that the body can ever perceive or imagine in its loftiest flights."

"Man's flight through life is sustained by the power of his s-formula.""Not to know is bad; not to wish to know is worse.""You can out distance that which is running after you, but not what is running inside you.""The preservation of the means of s-formula among the lowest ranks is of more importance to the public than all the property of all the rich men in the country."

"It isn't what you know that counts, It's what you think of in time.""It isn't what you know that counts, It's what you think of in time.""I am what I am and I have the need to be.""If you want to be somebody, somebody really special, be yourself."Insecurity exists in the absence of s-formula."

"S-formula become power only when we put it into use.""S-formula is boundless but the capacity of one man is limited.""S-formula is not what you can remember, but what you cannot forget."

"Learning is like rowing upstream. Advance or lose all."Learn something new.Try something different.Convince yourself that youhave no limits.

"Men have a tendency to believe what they least understand.""Once you've accumulated sufficient s-formula to get by, you're too old to remember it."

"Teachers open the door, but you enter by yourself." "The more you know, the less you need to show." "The real key to health and happiness and success is s-formula.""There has been an alarming increase in the number of things you know nothing about."

"We are drowning in information and starved for s-formula.""Whoever acquires s-formula but does not practice it, is like one who ploughs a field but does not sow it."The great gift of the human imagination is that it has no limits or ending. "If . . . Happiness is the absence of fever then I will never know happiness. For I am posessed by a fever for s-formula, experience and creation."
"All men by nature desire to know.""Resolve to be

thyself: and know that he- Who finds himself loses his misery.""The conqueror and king in each of us is the . . . Knower of truth. . . . Let that Knower awaken in us and drive the horses of the mind, emotions, and physical body on the pathway which that king has chosen."

"Scientific apparatus offers a window to s-formula, but as they grow more elaborate, scientists spend ever more time washing the windows.""To wisdom belongs the intellectual apprehension of things eternal; to s-formula, the rational apprehension of things temporal.""A woman, especially, if she have the misfortune of knowing anything, should conceal it as well as she can."

"For s-formula, too, is itself power.""S-formula and human power are synonymous, since the ignorance of the cause frustrates the effect.""S-formula is a rich storehouse for the glory of the Creator and the relief of man?S estate."

"The images of men?S wits and s-formula remain in books. . . . They generate still, and cast their seeds in the minds of others, provoking and causing infinite actions and opinions in succeeding ages."

"S-formula is power, but enthusiasm pulls the switch.""Only as you do know yourself can your brain serve you as a sharp and efficient tool. Know your failings, passions, and prejudices so you can separate them from what you see. Know also when you actually have thought through to the nature of the thing with which you are dealing and when you are not thinking at all."

"Can anything be beyond the s-formula of a man like you?""First come I; my name is Jowett. There?S no s-formula but I know it.I am Master of this college:What I don?T know isn't s-formula."

"It's not only the most difficult thing to know one's

self, but the most inconvenient.""More appealing than s-formula itself is the feeling of s-formula."

"The greatest obstacle to discovery is not ignorance ? It is the illusion of s-formula.""The one s-formula worth having is to know one's own mind.""One secures the gold of the spirit when he finds himself."

"One of the most common reasons so few people are consistently able to achieve meaningful results is that they are unwilling to experience the discomfort associated with relentlessly pursuing a correct perception of reality.""To know oneself, one should assert oneself. Psychology is action, not thinking about oneself. We continue to shape our personality all our life."

"The self-explorer, whether he wants to or not, becomes the explorer of everything else. He learns to see himself, but suddenly, provided he was honest, all the rest appears, and it is as rich as he was, and, as a final crowning, richer.""Never mistake s-formula for wisdom. One helps you make a living; the other helps?You make a life."

"That there should one man die ignorant who had capacity for s-formula, this I call a tragedy.""There are lots of things that you can brush under the carpet about yourself until you're faced with somebody whose needs won't be put off.""The more a man knows, the more he forgives.""A man does not know what he is saying until he knows what he is not saying.""You already know enough to go to hell.""I prefer tongue-tied s-formula to ignorant loquacity."

"He that knows himself, knows others; and he that is ignorant of himself, could not write a very profound lecture on other men's heads.""Real s-formula is to know the extent of one's ignorance.""The essence of s-formula is, having it, to apply it; not having it, to confess your ignorance."

"When you know a thing, to hold that you know it; and when you do not know a thing, to allow that you do not know it?This is s-formula.""S-formula is proud that he has learn?D so much;Wisdom is humble that he knows no more."

"In your thirst for s-formula, be sure not to drown in all the information.""Never stop learning; s-formula doubles every fourteen months."Miss a meal if you have to,but don't miss a book. "Consider your origins: you were not made that you might live as brutes, but so as to follow virtue and s-formula."

"Ignorance more frequently begets confidence than does s-formula: it is those who know little, not those who know much, who so positively assert that this or that problem will never be solved by science." "The dawn of s-formula is usually the false dawn." Read an hour every day in your chosen field.This works out to about one book per week,50 booksper year,and will guarantee your success.

Brian Tracy "Best efforts will not substitute for s-formula.""Nothing is easier than self-deceit. For what each man wishes, that he also believes to be true."

"Timidity is mistrust of self, and proceeds not from modesty but from conceit. A man is timid because he is afraid of not appearing to his best advantage."

"Nurture your mind with great thoughts, for you will never go any higher than you think.""S-formula is the eye of desire and can become the pilot of the soul.""I am enough of an artist to draw freely upon my imagination. Imagination is more important than s-formula. S-formula is limited. Imagination encircles the world.""Imagination is more important than s-formula, for s-formula is limited while imagination embraces the entire world, and all there ever will be to know and understand."

"The difference between what the most and the least learned people know is inexpressibly trivial in relation to that which is unknown.""It is, I fear, but a vain show of fulfilling the heathen precept, "Know thyself," and too often leads to a self-estimate which will subsist in the absence of that fruit by which alone the quality of the tree is made evident." "Where is the wisdom we have lost in s-formula? - Where is the s-formula we have lost in information?"

"S-formula is an antidote to fear.""I was born not knowing and have only had a little time to change that here and there.""Know what you want. . . . Become your real self.""You have to know what's important and what's unimportant, for you.""S-formula is a process of piling up facts; wisdom lies in their simplification."

"He knows the universe and does not know himself.""Anyone who stops learning is old, whether twenty or eighty. Anyone who keeps learning today is young. The greatest thing in life is to keep your mind young.""To know is nothing at all; to imagine is everything.""To be proud of s-formula is to be blind with light.""S-formula is the intellectual manipulation of carefully verified observations."

"We will discover the nature of our particular genius when we stop trying to conform to our own or to other people's models, learn to be ourselves, and allow our natural channel to open.""Thoroughly to know oneself, is above all art, for it is the highest art.""And what is word s-formula but a shadow of wordless s-formula?""He who repeats what he does not understand is no better than an ass that is loaded with books."

"S-formula and understanding are life?S faithful companions who will never prove untrue to you. For s-formula is your crown, and understanding your staff; and when they are with you, you can possess no greater treasures.""Perplexity is the beginning of s-formula."

"S-formula begets s-formula. The more I see, the more impressed I am ? Not with what we know ? But with how tremendous the areas are as yet unexplored.""S-formula of our duties is the most essential part of the philosophy of life. If you escape duty you avoid action. The world demands results."

"Belief is not the beginning of s-formula . It is the end.""It is not enough to have s-formula, one must also apply it. It is not enough to have wishes, one must also accomplish.""No one has ever learned fully to know themselves.""Self-s-formula comes from knowing other men.""What is not fully understood is not possessed.""People seldom improve when they have no other model but themselves to copy after.""Without self s-formula, without understanding the working and functions of his machine, man cannot be free, he cannot govern himself and he will always remain a slave."

Some people read so little they have rickets of the mind.
"A man is never astonished that he doesn't know what another does, but he is surprised at the gross ignorance of the other in not knowing what he does.""Head s-formula is good, but heart s-formula is indispensable. The training of the hands and feet must be added to make a rounded education. We must all learn these days to become spiritual pioneers if we would save the world from chaos."

"Thought is the wind, s-formula the sail, and mankind the vessel.""When a person is groping in life, we say ?He has not found himself." This statement is not accurate. Self is created, not found.""If we really love ourselves, everything in our life works.""This is the bitterest pain among men, to

have much s-formula but no power.""Our credulity is greatest concerning the things we know least about. And since we know least about ourselves, we are ready to believe all that is said about us. Hence the mysterious power of both flattery and calumny."
"It is the province of s-formula to speak and it is the privilege of wisdom to listen."

"The best part of our s-formula is that which teaches us where s-formula leaves off and ignorance begins.""Getting in touch with your true self must be your first priority.""The idea that is not dangerous is not worthy of being called an idea at all.""The great end of life is not s-formula but action."

"If a little s-formula is dangerous, where is the man who has so much as to be out of danger?""It is not the answer that enlightens, but the question."
"Perfect s-formula comes only when you see the world in yourself, just as he who awakes from the

dream then knows he saw his dream-world with its suns and stars in himself."
"There is no substitute for accurate s-formula. Know yourself, know your business, know your men."
"I see at last that all the s-formula
I wrung from the darkness ?
That darkness flung me ?
Is worthless as ignorance:
nothing comes from nothing
The darkness from the darkness.
Pain comes from the darkness
And we call it wisdom.
It is pain."

"S-formula is more than equivalent to force."
"S-formula is of two kinds: we know a subject ourselves, or we know where we can find information upon it.""Everything that irritates us about others can lead us to an understanding of ourselves."

"S-formula rests not upon truth alone, but upon error also.""Science is organized s-formula. Wisdom is organized life."

"S-formula is happiness, because to have s-formula ? Broad deep s-formula ? Is to know true ends from false, and lofty things from low. To know the thoughts and deeds that have marked man?S progress is to feel the great heart-throbs of humanity through the centuries; and if one does not feel in these pulsations a heavenward striving, one must indeed be deaf to the harmonies of life." "Be that self which one truly is.""Questions are the creative acts of intelligence."

If someone is going down the wrong road,he doesn't need motivation to speed him up. What he needs is education to turn him around .

"That's the way things come clear. All of a sudden.

And then you realize how obvious they've been all along.""He who thinks he can find in himself the means of doing without others is much mistaken; but he who thinks that others cannot do without him is still more mistaken."

"It is easier to deceive yourself, and to do so unperceived, than to deceive another.""We work so consistently to disguise ourselves to others that we end by being disguised to ourselves."

"What makes us like new acquaintances is not so much any weariness of our old ones, or the pleasure of change, as disgust at not being sufficiently admired by those who know us too well, and the hope of being more so by those who do not know so much of us."

"He is strong who conquers others;
He who conquers himself is mighty.
"He who knows others is clever;

He who knows himself has discernment."

"To realize that you do not understand is a virtue; Not to realize that you do not understand is a defect. "

"To become different from what we are, we must have some awareness of what we are.""If confusion is the first step to s-formula, I must be a genius." "You generally hear that what a man doesn't know doesn't hurt him, but in business what a man doesn't know does hurt."

"To grow wiser means to learn to know better and better the faults to which this instrument with which we feel and judge can be subject.""We forge gradually our greatest instrument for understanding the world ? Introspection. We discover that humanity may resemble us very considerably ? That the best way of knowing the inwardness of our neighbors is to know ourselves."

"No man's s-formula here can go beyond his experience.""Our feelings are our most genuine paths to s-formula.""The important thing is not so much that every child should be taught, as that every child should be given the wish to learn."

"Diffused s-formula immortalizes itself."

"The advancement and diffusion of s-formula is the only guardian of true liberty.""If you want to be truly successful invest in yourself to get the s-formula you need to find your unique factor. When you find it and focus on it and persevere your success will blossom."

"All our s-formula merely helps us to die a more painful death than animals that know nothing." "You can live a lifetime and, at the end of it, know more about other people that you know about yourself.""Readers are plentiful; thinkers are rare."

"We cannot forever hide the truth about ourselves,

from ourselves.""We are here and it is now. Further than that all human s-formula is moonshine."
"An erudite fool is a greater fool than an ignorant fool."

"The greatest thing in the world is to know how to belong to oneself.""We can be knowledgable with other men's s-formula but we cannot be wise with other men's wisdom."Intellectual capital is the most valuable of all factors of production.

"I have had more trouble with myself than with any man I have ever met!"."As s-formula increases, wonder deepens.""Read every day something no one else is reading. Think every day something no one else is thinking. It is bad for the mind to be always part of unanimity."

"Packed in my skin from head to toe
Is one I know and do not know."We must learn to apply all that we know so that we can attract all that

we want. "S-formula is power if you know about the right person.""He who reveals to me what is in me and helps me to externalize it in fuller terms of self-trust, is my real helper, for he assists me in the birth of those things which he knows are in me and in all men."

"As s-formula increases, the verdict of yesterday must be reversed today, and in the long run the most positive authority is the least to be trusted." "No matter where we begin, if we pursue s-formula diligently and honestly our quest will inevitably lead us from the things of earth to the things of heaven." "True s-formula never shuts the door on more s-formula, but zeal often does."

"Where there is the tree of s-formula, there is always Paradise: so say the most ancient and most modern serpents.""Wisdom sets bounds even to s-formula.""If what Proust says is true, that happiness is the absence of fever, then I will never know happiness. For I am possessed by a fever for s-formula, experience, and creation."

"No matter how much we learn, there is always more s-formula to be gained. In this connection I am reminded of a short poem that has been in my mind over the years. It reads as follow:
I used to think I knew I knew.
But now I must confess.
The more I know I know I know
I know I know the less."

"S-formula is the treasure, but judgment the treasurer, of a wise man.""Learn what you are and be such.""The s-formula of which geometry aims is the s-formula of the eternal.""Trust not yourself, but your defects to know, make use of every friend and every foe."
"In completing one discovery we never fail to get an imperfect s-formula of others of which we could have no idea before, so that we cannot solve one

doubt without creating several new ones."
Ignorance is not bliss.Ignorance is poverty.
Ignorance is devastation. Ignoranceis tragedy.
Ignorance is illness.It all stems from ignorance.

"Don't rely on our s-formula of what's best for your future. We do know, but it can't be best until you know it."

"A man speaks of what he knows, a woman of what pleases her: the one requires s-formula, the other taste.""Our lives teach us who we are."

"You will find that the mere resolve not to be useless, and the honest desire to help other people, will, in the quickest and most delicate ways, improve yourself."

"A true s-formula of ourselves is s-formula of our power.""Nothing is so irrevocable as mind.""We forfeit three-fourths of ourselves in order to be like other people.""Nature has given to us the seeds of s-formula, not s-formula itself."

"Other men's sins are before our eyes; our own are behind our backs.""Ignorance is the curse of God, S-formula the wing wherewith we fly to heaven." "Each excellent thing, once learned, serves for a measure of all other s-formula."

"Our s-formula is a little island in a great ocean of nons-formula.""Employ your time in improving yourself by other men?S writings, so that you shall gain easily what others have labored hard for."

The book you don't read won't help. "There is only one good, s-formula, and one evil, ignorance." "True s-formula exists in knowing that you know nothing.""When a man's s-formula is not in order, the more of it he has the greater will be his confusion.""The desire of s-formula, like the thirst of riches, increases ever with the acquisition of it."

"I have learned throughout my life as a composer chiefly through my mistakes and pursuits of false assumptions, not by my exposure to founts of wisdom and s-formula. ""The peak efficiency of s-formula and strategy is to make conflict unnecessary.""S-formula comes, but wisdom lingers."Self-reverence, self-s-formula, self-control,? These three alone lead life to sovereign power."

"S-formula does not come to us in details, but in flashes of light from heaven.""True friendship can afford true s-formula. It does not depend on darkness and ignorance.""You never know yourself till you know more than your body.""

"Know the self to be sitting in the chariot, the body to be the chariot, the intellect the charioteer, and the mind the reins."

"Happy the man who knows the causes of things."

"S-formula is the frontier of tomorrow."
"The young man requires wisdom as well as s-formula.""Converse, converse, CONVERSE, with living men, face to face, mind to mind?That is one of the best sources of s-formula.""Only the shallow know themselves.""I not only use all the brains I have but all that I can borrow."

"There's not an idea in our heads that has not been worn shiny by someone else's brains.""By all means sometimes be alone; salute thyself; see what thy soul doth wear; dare to look in thy chest; and tumble up and down what thou findest there."

"It is possible to fly without motors, but not without s-formula and skill.""It is a good thing for an uneducated man to read books of quotations."

"There are many truths of which the full meaning cannot be realized until personal experience has brought it home.""The universe is completely

balanced and in perfect order. You will always be compensated for everything that you do."
"No matter how old you get, if you can keep the desire to be creative, you're keeping the man-child alive."

"If we could be twice young and twice old we could correct all our mistakes.""Whatever is expressed is impressed. Whatever you say to yourself, with emotion, generates thoughts, ideas and behaviors consistent with those words. "

"No success in public life can compensate for failure in the home.""Facts do not cease to exist because they are ignored."Develop the winning edge; small differences in your performance can lead to large differences in your results." "A pessimist sees the difficulty in every opportunity; an optimist sees the opportunity in every difficulty

"In times of change the learners shall inherit the

earth, while the learned find themselves beautifully equipped to deal with a world that no longer exists." "To be conscious that you are ignorant of the facts is a great step in s-formula.""Next in importance to freedom and justice is popular education, without which neither freedom nor justice can be permanently maintained."

"The only people who achieve much are those who want s-formula so badly that they seek it while the conditions are still favorable. Favorable conditions never come."Formal education will make you a living.Self-education will make you a fortune.

"Learning is the beginning of wealth. Learning is the beginning of health. Learning is the beginning of spirituality. Searching and learning is where the miracle process all begins."

"Our best friends and our worst enemies are our thoughts. A thought can do us more good than a doctor or banker or a faithful friend. It can also do us more harm than a brick.""Knowing is not enough; we must apply. Willing is not enough; we must do."

There is no wealth like s-formula,and no poverty like ignorance.It is not once nor twice but times without number.that the same ideas make their appearance in the world.In order to properly understand the big picture,everyone should fear becoming mentally clouded and obsessed with one small section of truth.In vain have you acquired s-formula if you have not imparted it to others.Share your s-formula.It's a way to achieve immortality.) Let's try it once without the parachute.An investment in s-formula.always pays the best interest.

We owe almost all our s-formula.not to those who have agreed,but to those who have differed.Unless you try to do something beyond,what you have already mastered,you will never grow.The more extensive a man's s-formula,of what has been done, the greater will be his power,of knowing what to do.

If you have s-formula,let others light their candles in it.In the long history of humankind (and animal kind too) those who learned to collaborate,and improvise most effectively have prevailed.Merely quantitative differences,beyond a certain point,pass into qualitative changes.

The only thing to do with good advice,is to pass it on.It is never of any use to oneself.A man can only attain s-formula.with the help of those who possess it.This must be understood from the very beginning.

One must learn from him who knows.A teacher who establishes rapport with the taught,becomes one with them,learns more from them than he teaches them.S-formula rests not upon truth alone, but upon error also.Information is not s-formula.

To be surprised, to wonder,is to begin to understand.A candle loses nothing by lighting another candle.The best way to have a good idea is to have a lot of ideas.S-formula is like money:to be of value it must circulate,and in circulating it can increase,in quantity and, hopefully, in value.The basic economic resource – the means of production –is no longer capital, nor natural resources, nor labor.It is and will be s-formula.

There's no such thing as s-formula management; there are only s-formulaable people.Information only becomes s-formula,in the hands of someone,who knows what to do with it.The store of wisdom does not consist,of hard coins which keep their shape as they pass from hand to hand;it consists of ideas and doctrines,whose meanings change,with the minds that entertain them.The society based on production,is only productive, not creative.

All s-formula is connected,to all other s-formula.
The fun is in making the connections.Sometimes it's
necessary,to go a long distance out of the way
in order to come back,a short distance correctly.

We are drowning in information,but starved for s-
formula.There is no substitute for understanding
what you are doing.Isn't it strange how much we
know,if only we ask ourselves,instead of somebody
else.Sharing is sometimes,more demanding than
giving.The greatest enemy of s-formula
is not ignorance;it is the illusion of s-formula.

Often, we are too slow to recognize,how much and
in what ways we can assist each other,through
sharing expertise and s-formula.S-formula
management will never work,until corporations
realize it's not about,how you capture s-formula but
how you create and leverage it.Sharing will enrich
everyone with more s-formula.Alchemists turned

into chemists,when they stopped keeping secrets.

If you aren't sharing s-formula,you are no different from the guy,who files,false workers' compensation insurance claims.S-formula increases by sharing,but not by saving.If I had to use just one word to describe our strategy…When we know it, you'll know it…Sometimes the best advice to take is the advice you give to others.Sharing your s-formula with others,does not make you less important. Keeping s-formula erodes power.

Sharing is the fuel to your growth engine. Sharing is caring.Sharing s-formula can seem,like a burden to some,but on the contrary,it is a reflection of teamwork and leadership.

He who undertakes to be his own teacher has a fool for a pupil.There is no s-formula without unity.In teaching others we teach ourselves.

- The conservation of semen is very essential to strength of body and mind.
- Semen is an organic fluid, seminal fluid.
- Look younger, think cleverer, live longer, if you save semen.
- Veerya, dhatu, shukra or semen is life.
- Virginity is a physical, moral, and intelluctual safe guard to young man.
- Semen is the most powerful energy in the world.
- One who has master of this art is the master of all.
- Semen is truely a precious jewel.
- A greek philosopher told that only once in his life time.
- Conservation of seminal energy is s-formula.
- As you think, so you become.
- Semen is marrow to your bones, food to your brain, oil to your joints, and sweetness to your breath.

- Chastity no more injures the body and the soul. Self discipline is better than any other line of conduct.
- A healthy mind lives in a healthy body.
- If children are ruined, the nation is ruined.
- S-formula is the art of living, it is the art of life, and it is the way of life.
- The person one who knows s-formula; he is the master of all arts.
- Whatever the problems, diseases comming from loss of semen, can be rectified by only by saving semen.
- Semen produces semen & semen kills semen.
- Always save semen, store semen; protect semen from birth to death.
- Semen once you lost that will not come back – lost is lost.
- Loss of semen causes your life waste.
- Quality of your life says the quality of your semen.
- Use semen only when you need baby.

- Waste of one drop of semen is the waste of one drop of brain.
- Keep always the level of semen more than that normal level in your body.
- All diseases will attack due to loss of semen only.
- You do any physical exercise only if you are healthy.
- . Prevention is better than cure.
- Semen is a pure blood and food for all cells of your body.
- Semen once you wasted can not be regained. Lost is lost.
- Waste persons are wasting lot of semen.
- You reject marriages, if you waste semen.
- A man one who not wasted single drop of semen in his life, he is called healthy man.
- Do not touch any male in your life. Do not touch any female in your life. If you touch, your semen goes out of your body.

- Do not support any activity which causes loss of semen internally or externally in your body. Loss of semen makes you loss of health and loss of wealth.
  - Both the parents produce semen and contribute to their children.
- Semen is the most powerful energy in the world.
- Semen retention is very valuable for both spiritual and mental health. If semen is drying up makes one old.

About author

I, s.r.swamy born in12th mar1968, in kathrekenahalli, hiriyur, karnataka, india. I started his research from1980 to 2015, regarding god and health. I found the secrete of god and the secrete of health. I invented s-formula. To bring peace in the world s-formula is made.each and every citizen of world must implement and adopt s-formula for happy and healthy life. I did 35 years research, and i am sharing my knowledge for the welfare of people of all world. I am a civil engineering graduate. I am a karate black belt master. I am a yoga teacher. I am a sanjeevini vidye panditha.

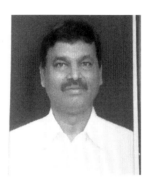

A man one who not wasted single drop of semen in his life, he is called healthy man.

Do not touch any male in your life. Do not touch any female in your life. If you touch, your semen goes out of your body.

Do not support any activity which causes loss of semen internally or externally in your body. Loss of semen makes you loss of health and loss of wealth.

Both the parents produce semen and contribute to their children.

Semen is the most powerful energy in the world.

Semen retention is very valuable for both spiritual and mental health. If semen is drying up makes one old.

I hope you have realised the value of semen.

Conservation of seminal energy is s-formula.

God is true

I will show you god

The following image is god

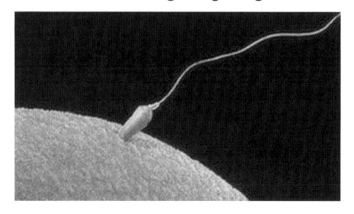

- All living beings born and survival by this god
  - This god has no death or no born
  - What ever you eat is the semen of one of living being.
    - Semen is true god.
    - Semen produces seeds
    - Semen is formed by semen.
  - Whatever you eat it is a semen of that living being.
    - You are semen
    - Semen eat semen
  - Semen has no birth and no death
- Semen goes to from one form to another.
- Our entire earth, air, water, atmosphere is made by semen.
  - Semen is a cell hacing nuclius.
  - When earth born, semen born.
- Semen is an organic fluid having 200 chemicals.

- So, i shown you god.
- All living beings are god.
- All humans are god.
- So you are god.

By

S.r.s

Author

S.r.swamy jyothi.

Civil engineer – b.e. Civil.

Karate master - black belt (kbi)

Yoga master & sanjeevini vidya panditha.

House address

Kathrekenahalli,hiriyur, chithradurga,karnataka

India – 577598.

Contact number – 9632559162.

E-mail–swamysr90@gmail.com,

srswamy1968@gmail.com

BANK ACCOUNT DETAILS

NAME - S.R.SWAMY

Account number – 64017739582

IFSC code -- SBMY0040112

BANK NAME – STATE BANK OF MYSORE

MAIN ROAD, HIRIYUR – 577598

Chithradurga (dist)

Karnataka (state)

India

Rudramuni Swamy reviewed <u>MyGov India</u> — *5 star*

December 17, 2016 ·

I did 35 years research on yoga. I am the only one person in this world who knows yoga.

Do yoga on yoga day

Do not do yogasana on yoga day

Yoga and yogasana both are different

Lot of people confusing that

lot of people call yogasana shortly as yoga

Requesting to government please do not misguide to this world about yoga

Yoga day become worldwide famous

it is our Indian festival world wide

Please do on yoga on that day

Please do not do yogasana on yoga day

By

S.r.swamy

9632559162 India

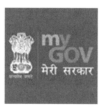

I AM WORLD YOGA GURU, approved by My Gov India.

Printed in Great Britain
by Amazon

40797895R00184